Electromyography

Editor

DEVON I. RUBIN

NEUROLOGIC CLINICS

www.neurologic.theclinics.com

Consulting Editor
RANDOLPH W. EVANS

November 2021 • Volume 39 • Number 4

ELSEVIER

1600 John F. Kennedy Boulevard • Suite 1800 • Philadelphia, Pennsylvania, 19103-2899

http://www.theclinics.com

NEUROLOGIC CLINICS Volume 39, Number 4
November 2021 ISSN 0733-8619, ISBN-13: 978-0-323-77941-8

Editor: Stacy Eastman
Developmental Editor: Hannah Almira Lopez

Neurologic Clinics (ISSN 0733-8619) is published quarterly by Elsevier Inc., 360 Park Avenue South, New York, NY 10010–1710. Months of issue are February, May, August, and November. Periodicals postage paid at New York, NY, and additional mailing offices. Subscription prices are $333.00 per year for US individuals, $881.00 per year for US institutions, $100.00 per year for US students, $408.00 per year for Canadian individuals, $938.00 per year for Canadian institutions, $461.00 per year for international individuals, $938.00 per year for international institutions, $210.00 for foreign students/residents, and $100.00 for Canadian students/residents. To receive student/resident rate, orders must be accompanied by name of affiliated institution, date of term, and the *signature* of program/residency coordinator on institution letterhead. Orders will be billed at individual rate until proof of status is received. Foreign air speed delivery is included in all *Clinics* subscription prices. All prices are subject to change without notice. **POSTMASTER:** Send address changes to *Neurologic Clinics*, Elsevier Health Sciences Division, Subscription Customer Service, 3251 Riverport Lane, Maryland Heights, MO 63043. **Customer Service: Telephone: 1-800-654-2452 (U.S. and Canada); 314-447-8871 (outside U.S. and Canada). Fax: 314-447-8029. E-mail: journalscustomerservice-usa@elsevier.com (for print support); journalsonlinesupport-usa@elsevier.com (for online support).**

Reprints. For copies of 100 or more of articles in this publication, please contact the Commercial Reprints Department, Elsevier Inc., 360 Park Avenue South, New York, New York, 10010-1710; Tel.: +1-212-633-3874; Fax: +1-212-633-3820, and E-mail: reprints@elsevier.com.

Neurologic Clinics is also published in Spanish by Nueva Editorial Interamericana S.A., Mexico City, Mexico.

Neurologic Clinics is covered in *Current Contents/Clinical Medicine, MEDLINE/PubMed (Index Medicus), EMBASE/Excerpta Medica, and PsycINFO, and ISI/BIOMED.*

Contributors

CONSULTING EDITOR

RANDOLPH W. EVANS, MD
Clinical Professor, Department of Neurology, Baylor College of Medicine, Houston, Texas, USA

EDITOR

DEVON I. RUBIN, MD
Professor, Department of Neurology, Director, EMG Laboratory, Mayo Clinic, Jacksonville, Florida, USA

AUTHORS

ALON ABRAHAM, MD
Neuromuscular Diseases Unit, Department of Neurology, Tel Aviv Sourasky Medical Center, Tel Aviv, Israel

JEFFREY S. CALVIN, MD
Department of Neurology, Clinical Neurophysiology Fellow, Saint Louis University School of Medicine, St Louis, Missouri, USA

PRIYA SAI DHAWAN, MD, FRCPC
Assistant Professor, Department of Neurology, University of British Columbia, Vancouver, British Columbia, Canada

TAYLOR B. HARRISON, MD
Associate Professor, Department of Neurology, Emory University School of Medicine, Atlanta, Georgia, USA

GHAZALA HAYAT, MD
Professor of Neurology, Saint Louis University School of Medicine, St Louis, Missouri, USA

HOLLI A. HORAK, MD
Professor of Neurology, University of College of Medicine - Tucson, Tucson, Arizona, USA

SPENCER K. HUTTO, MD
Assistant Professor, Department of Neurology, Emory University School of Medicine, Atlanta, Georgia, USA

XUAN KANG, MD
Assistant Professor, Department of Neurology, University of Colorado Denver, Aurora, Colorado, USA

HANS D. KATZBERG, MD, MSc, FRCPC
Division of Neurology, University Health Network, Toronto General Hospital, Toronto, Ontario, Canada

JOHN KINCAID, MD
Department of Neurology, Indiana University School of Medicine, IU Health Neuroscience Center, Indianapolis, Indiana, USA

CHRISTOPHER J. LAMB, MD
Department of Neurology, Mayo Clinic, Jacksonville, Florida, USA

KERRY H. LEVIN, MD
Professor of Neurology, Cleveland Clinic Lerner College of Medicine, Chairman, Department of Neurology, Cleveland Clinic, Cleveland, Ohio, USA

ROBERT J. MARQUARDT, DO
Clinical Assistant Professor of Neurology, Neuromuscular Center, Department of Neurology, Cleveland Clinic, Cleveland, Ohio, USA

JENNIFER M. MARTINEZ-THOMPSON, MD
Assistant Professor, Department of Neurology, Mayo Clinic, Rochester, Minnesota, USA

REBECCA O'BRYAN, MD
Department of Physical Medicine and Rehabilitation, Indiana University School of Medicine, IU Health Neuroscience Center, Indianapolis, Indiana, USA

KAMAKSHI PATEL, MD
University of Texas Medical Branch (UTMB), Galveston, Texas, USA

DIANNA QUAN, MD
Professor, Department of Neurology, University of Colorado Denver, Aurora, Colorado, USA

DEVON I. RUBIN, MD
Professor, Department of Neurology, Director, EMG Laboratory, Mayo Clinic, Jacksonville, Florida, USA

ROCIO VAZQUEZ DO CAMPO, MD
Assistant Professor, Department of Neurology, The University of Alabama at Birmingham, Birmingham, Alabama, USA

Contents

Preface: Practical Concepts in Electromyography   ix

Devon I. Rubin

Nerve Conduction Studies: Basic Concepts and Patterns of Abnormalities   897

Rebecca O'Bryan and John Kincaid

> Nerve conduction studies are a key component of the electrophysiologic evaluation of the peripheral nerve system, and provide important information about the integrity of the large, myelinated axons, neuromuscular junctions, and muscle. Nerve conduction studies involve eliciting nerve action potentials at sites along a peripheral nerve and recording the response from another site along the nerve or from a muscle innervated by that nerve. Attention to details of test performance, use of well-established normative values, and knowledge of the patterns of abnormality produced by disorders that affect neuronal, axonal, and myelin sheath function are fundamental for proper interpretation of results.

Needle Electromyography Waveforms During Needle Electromyography   919

Devon I. Rubin

> Needle electromyography (EMG) waveforms recorded during needle EMG help to define the type, temporal course, and severity of a neuromuscular disorder. Accurate interpretation of EMG waveforms is a critical component of an electrodiagnostic examination. This article reviews the significance of spontaneous EMG waveforms and changes in voluntary motor unit potentials in neuromuscular disorders.

Electrodiagnosis of Common Mononeuropathies: Median, Ulnar, and Fibular (Peroneal) Neuropathies   939

Kamakshi Patel and Holli A. Horak

> This article addresses common mononeuropathies seen in the electrodiagnostic laboratory. The most common mononeuropathies—median neuropathy at the wrist (carpal tunnel syndrome), ulnar neuropathy at the elbow, and fibular (peroneal) neuropathy at the fibular head—are reviewed. The causes, clinical presentations, approached to the electrodiagnostic studies (including nerve conduction studies and needle electromyography), and the typical findings are discussed.

Electrodiagnostic Assessment of Uncommon Mononeuropathies   957

Ghazala Hayat and Jeffrey S. Calvin

> Carpal tunnel syndrome, ulnar neuropathy at the elbow, and peroneal neuropathy are the most common mononeuropathies; however, other individual nerves may also be injured by various processes. These uncommon mononeuropathies may be less readily diagnosed owing to unfamiliarity with the presentations and vague symptoms. Electrodiagnostic studies

are essential in the evaluation of uncommon mononeuropathies and can assist in localization and prognostication. However, they can also be challenging; stimulation at the proximal sites is difficult and well-validated reference values are not available. This article reviews the electrodiagnostic assessment of several uncommon upper and lower extremities mononeuropathies.

Electrodiagnostic Assessment of Radiculopathies   983

Robert J. Marquardt and Kerry H. Levin

This article discusses the electrodiagnostic assessment of radiculopathy. Relevant anatomy initially is reviewed followed by discussion surrounding the approach to nerve conduction studies and needle electrode examination when it comes to radiculopathy evaluation. Pitfalls of the electrodiagnosis versus clinical diagnosis of radiculopathy and the definitions of acute versus chronic, and active versus inactive, are reviewed.

Electrodiagnostic Assessment of Plexopathies   997

Priya Sai Dhawan

Disorders of the brachial and lumbosacral plexus are complex and may occur as a consequence of trauma, compression, inflammatory disorders, malignant infiltration, or delayed effects of radiation therapy. An understanding of plexus anatomy and surrounding structures will allow the electromyographer to facilitate an efficient and comprehensive assessment of the plexus. A careful and thorough electrodiagnostic assessment allows for localization within the plexus and may provide important information about underlying pathology and prognosis.

Electrodiagnostic Assessment of Polyneuropathy   1015

Rocio Vazquez Do Campo

This article focuses on principles of nerve conduction studies and needle electromyography applied to the electrodiagnosis of polyneuropathy. The components of the electrodiagnostic evaluation of polyneuropathy and the electrophysiological characteristics of axonal and demyelinating neuropathies and nodo-paranodopathies are reviewed.

Electrodiagnostic Assessment of Myopathy   1035

Jennifer M. Martinez-Thompson

 Video content accompanies this article at http://www.neurologic. theclinics.com.

Electrodiagnostic testing is a useful tool in the evaluation of suspected myopathy and helps to confirm the presence of a myopathy and exclude disease mimickers. The electrodiagnostic pattern of findings during testing guides subsequent laboratory evaluation, genetic testing, and in identifying potential muscle biopsy targets. It also provides a baseline for subsequent assessment of disease progression or response to therapy. This article summarizes the approach to electrodiagnostic assessment in various myopathic disorders.

Electrodiagnostic Assessment of Neuromuscular Junction Disorders   1051

Hans D. Katzberg and Alon Abraham

Please verify edits, "These techniques", or specify. This article reviews advanced electrodiagnostic techniques used to assess for neuromuscular junction disorders, including repetitive nerve stimulation, conventional or concentric-needle single-fiber electromyography (SFEMG), and stimulated SFEMG. These techniques have high sensitivity but limited specificity. Novel methods currently under investigation are discussed, including vestibular ocular myogenic potential and oculography analysis.

Electrodiagnostic Assessment of Motor Neuron Disease   1071

Xuan Kang and Dianna Quan

Motor neuron diseases involve degeneration of motor neurons in the brain (upper motor neurons), brain stem, and spinal cord (lower motor neurons). Symptoms vary depending on the degree of upper and lower neuron involvement, but progressive painless weakness is the predominant complaint. Motor neuron disease includes numerous specific disorders, including amyotrophic lateral sclerosis, spinal muscular atrophy, spinal bulbar muscular atrophy, and other inherited and acquired conditions. Abnormalities on nerve conduction studies, repetitive nerve stimulation, needle electromyography, and other electrodiagnostic techniques help to distinguish these disorders from each other, and from other disorders with progressive weakness.

Electrodiagnostic Assessment of Hyperexcitable Nerve Disorders   1083

Spencer K. Hutto and Taylor B. Harrison

Peripheral nerve hyperexcitability (PNH) typically presents with complaints of muscle twitching, cramps, and muscle stiffness. Symptoms and signs indicating central and/or autonomic nervous system dysfunction also may be reported. An electroclinical spectrum exists, spanning from the milder cramp-fasciculation syndrome to more severe syndromes characterized by continuous muscle fiber activity. It is important to recognize that PNH may be an autoimmune phenomenon associated with antibodies targeting proteins of the voltage-gated potassium channel–complex and, in some patients, a paraneoplastic phenomenon. Symptomatic therapies include medicines that reduce neuronal excitability and in severe disease immunomodulatory treatments may be indicated.

Electromyography Case Examples: Practical Approaches to Neuromuscular Symptoms   1097

Christopher J. Lamb and Devon I. Rubin

Many neuromuscular complaints are evaluated with electrodiagnostic testing. In practice, physicians must plan the electrodiagnostic study to provide the most useful information addressing patients' symptoms. The approach to each study must be individualized based on the symptoms and findings of each previous result. This article reviews five real cases with common reasons for referral to the neurophysiology laboratory with discussion of the approach to testing, interpretation of the results, and practical decision-making points relevant to each case. The goal is to provide rationale for why specific studies were selected and how each was helpful in deriving the final diagnosis.

NEUROLOGIC CLINICS

FORTHCOMING ISSUES

February 2022
Hospital Neurology
Vanja C. Douglas and Maulik Shah, *Editors*

May 2022
Neurosurgery for Neurologists
Russell R. Lonser and Daniel K. Resnick, *Editors*

August 2022
Imaging of Headache
Sangam Kanekar, Editor

RECENT ISSUES

August 2021
Pediatric Neurology
Gary D. Clark, James J. Riviello, *Editors*

May 2021
Neurologic Emergencies
Joseph D. Burns and Anna M. Cervantes-Arslanian, *Editors*

February 2021
Therapy in Neurology
Jose Biller, *Editor*

ISSUES OF RELATED INTEREST

Neurosurgery Clinics
https://www.neurosurgery.theclinics.com/
Neuroimaging Clinics
https://www.neuroimaging.theclinics.com/
Psychiatric Clinics
https://www.psych.theclinics.com/
Child and Adolescent Psychiatric Clinics
https://www.childpsych.theclinics.com/

THE CLINICS ARE AVAILABLE ONLINE!
Access your subscription at:
www.theclinics.com

Preface

Practical Concepts in Electromyography

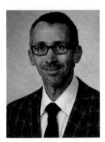

Devon I. Rubin, MD
Editor

Electromyography has been a longstanding valuable technique in the evaluation of neuromuscular disorders. The basic concepts of nerve conduction studies and needle electromyography were well established decades ago. While these same concepts still form the basis of the technique and interpretation of the studies today, advances in the techniques, approaches, and findings recorded during testing have helped physicians more accurately identify diseases. Furthermore, while advances in other ancillary testing, such as genetic testing and neuroimaging, have provided useful methods to diagnose neuromuscular disorders, electrodiagnostic testing provides information regarding the actual function of the neuromuscular system that cannot be assessed by other tests. This issue reviews the basic concepts of nerve conduction studies and needle electromyography and discusses the approaches and findings in different types of focal (common and uncommon mononeuropathies, radiculopathies) and generalized (motor neuron disorders, peripheral neuropathies, neuromuscular junction disorders, and myopathies) neuromuscular conditions. The goal of this issue is to provide the reader with a concise, practical reference that can be used to guide an understanding of the utility and limitation of electrodiagnostic testing in these disorders and to provide a guide for interpreting the findings in different conditions. An article dedicated to real examples encountered in the electromyography laboratory helps to

Neurol Clin 39 (2021) ix–x
https://doi.org/10.1016/j.ncl.2021.06.001
0733-8619/21/© 2021 Published by Elsevier Inc.

neurologic.theclinics.com

review approaches to specific patients and discusses the unique features of specific cases.

Devon I. Rubin, MD
Professor, Department of Neurology
Director, EMG Laboratory
Mayo Clinic

E-mail address:
Rubin.devon@mayo.edu

Nerve Conduction Studies
Basic Concepts and Patterns of Abnormalities

Rebecca O'Bryan, MD[a], John Kincaid, MD[b],*

KEYWORDS

- Nerve conduction studies • Electromyography • EMG • Electrophysiology

KEY POINTS

- The basic concepts of NCS are presented.
- The set ups for standard motor, sensory, mixed nerve and late response NCS are illustrated.
- The patterns of NCS abnormality encountered in neuronal, axonal and demyelinating lesions are presented.
- Technical issues impacting the reliability and reproducibility of NCS are discussed and illustrated.

INTRODUCTION

Nerve conduction studies (NCS) are one of the two primary components (along with needle electromyography [EMG]) of an electrodiagnostic evaluation for evaluating the neuromuscular system. NCS involve eliciting nerve action potentials at sites along a peripheral nerve and recording the response from another site along the nerve or from a muscle innervated by that nerve. NCS quantitatively evaluate the integrity of large, myelinated motor and sensory axons, and the neuromuscular junctions and the muscles. Small myelinated and unmyelinated axons are not assessed by standard NCS. An understanding of the factors related to nerve stimulation and recording, the meaning of the responses recorded, and technical factors that impact NCS are critical to the reliable performance and interpretation of the studies.

BASIC CONCEPTS OF STIMULATION

During NCS, action potentials in the peripheral axons are elicited by electrical stimuli delivered to the skin surface over the nerve, although needle electrodes are

[a] Department of Physical Medicine and Rehabilitation, Indiana University School of Medicine, IU Health Neuroscience Center, 355 W. 16th Street, Suite 3800, Indianapolis, IN 46202, USA;
[b] Department of Neurology, Indiana University School of Medicine, IU Health Neuroscience Center, 355 West 16th Street, Suite 4700, Indianapolis, IN 46202, USA
* Corresponding author.
E-mail address: jkincaid@iupui.edu

Neurol Clin 39 (2021) 897–917
https://doi.org/10.1016/j.ncl.2021.06.002
0733-8619/21/© 2021 Elsevier Inc. All rights reserved.

neurologic.theclinics.com

occasionally used. A bipolar stimulator is most common; the cathode is the source of depolarizing current and the anode collects the returning current and hyperpolarizes the underlying portion of the nerve. Depolarization of the axons to the threshold for action potential initiation is accomplished by direct current square wave pulses of 0.05 to 1.0 milliseconds duration. The strength of the depolarizing stimuli is quantified in voltage or amperage.

At each stimulation site, as the stimulus intensity is gradually increased, more axons are depolarized and the amplitude of the recorded waveform (which represents the summation of individual nerve or muscle fiber action potentials) increases and eventually reaches a maximum (**Fig. 1**). The stimulus intensity is increased by another 10% to 20% greater than maximum, to ensure that all axons within the nerve have been depolarized.

BASIC CONCEPTS OF RECORDING

Responses elicited from nerve stimulation are recorded from the skin surface over the nerve or muscle being studied using a three-electrode montage: E1 (black), E2 (red), and E0 (green) (**Fig. 2**).[1,2] The electrodes are connected to a preamplifier, and the difference in the electrical potential between the E1 and E2 electrodes is determined by a differential amplifier and displayed on the screen for analysis. The two recording electrodes are referred to as E1 and E2 (traditionally termed grid [G]1 and grid [G]2). The E0 electrode (traditionally referred to as the ground) serves as an electrical reference rather than being the zero or ground potential of an electrical circuit. The convention that a negative voltage at the E1 input produces an upward deflection on the instrument's display was adopted from that of electroencephalography during the formative years of EMG.

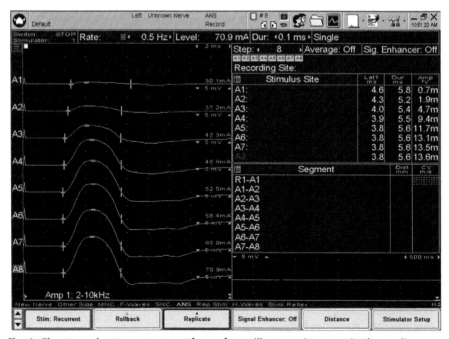

Fig. 1. The top to bottom sequence of waveforms illustrates increases in the median compound muscle action potential amplitude as stimulus strength is increased until a maximal response is produced. Stimulus strength is shown at the right end of each trace.

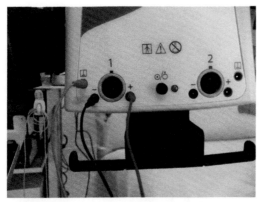

Fig. 2. The electrodes E1 (*black*), E2 (*red*), and E0 (*green*) connection into an EMG instrument amplifier.

TYPES OF NERVE CONDUCTION STUDIES

There are several types of NCS (motor, sensory, and mixed), which reflect the types of axons that are studied. Although the overall techniques are similar, there are important differences in meaning of the responses recorded.

Motor Nerve Conduction Studies

Motor NCS are performed by stimulating a nerve trunk and recording the response from a muscle supplied by that nerve. Because one motor axon innervates multiple muscle fibers and multiple motor units are present in a muscle, the recorded response is a summated response termed the compound muscle action potential (CMAP) or the M wave. The E1 electrode is located on the muscle belly over the motor point and E2 on the tendon (belly-tendon montage) (**Fig. 3**). The motor point is the site of clustering of neuromuscular junctions along the muscle and is the location that has the lowest stimulus threshold for producing a muscle twitch during faradaic stimulation in classical electrodiagnostic techniques. The tendon site of E2 was traditionally (and incorrectly) considered to be electrically inactive. In fact, in nerves, such as the ulnar and posterior tibial, the E2 electrode detects more activity than E1.[3,4] Although intramuscular concentric needles are used to record the responses from the muscle, they only record activity near the needle tip and the responses are not as reliable or reproducible as with surface electrodes. Common settings for motor NCS are listed in **Box 1**.

Motor NCS are used to test the integrity of the peripheral motor system, including the anterior horn cells, roots, peripheral nerves, neuromuscular junctions, and muscle. Abnormalities at each of these sites may impact the responses. For example, low CMAP amplitudes may occur in motor neuron diseases, polyradiculopathies, severe neuromuscular junction disorders, or myopathies. Thus, motor NCS alone are often insufficient to make a specific neuromuscular diagnosis. The complimentary information from sensory NCS and needle EMG are necessary for complete electrodiagnostic (EDX) interpretation. **Tables 1** and **2** list commonly and uncommonly performed motor NCS. Specifics of technique are available in standard EMG textbooks.[7,8]

Sensory Nerve Conduction Studies

Sensory NCS assess the integrity of the peripheral sensory axons. The responses recorded, termed the sensory nerve action potential (SNAP), are the summated action

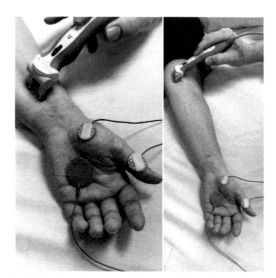

Fig. 3. Median motor NCS setup demonstrating recording electrodes over the muscle belly (E1) and tendon (E2), and ground electrode (E0) on the palm. The stimulator is shown at wrist and elbow stimulation sites. The stimulator tip closest to the recording electrodes is the cathode.

potentials of the large myelinated sensory axons within the nerve. Sensory responses are much lower in amplitude (microvolts) than CMAPs (millivolts). Stimulation methods are similar to motor NCS. Recording is performed using surface electrodes for most nerves, although deeper sensory nerves (eg, lateral femoral cutaneous nerve) may necessitate a needle recording electrode to obtain a reliable response. The E1 and E2 recording electrodes are both placed over the nerve, separated by approximately 4 cm for optimal amplitude resolution. E0 is placed between the stimulating and recording electrodes. Recording electrodes placed closer together than the width of the propagating action potential do not accurately capture the propagating activity, and electrodes placed too far apart produce a multiphasic waveform based on different arrival times of the action potential at E1 and E2. Sensory NCS settings are listed in **Box 2**.

NCS is reliably performed using an orthodromic or antidromic method. In the orthodromic method, a nerve is stimulated at a distal site (eg, using ring electrodes on a digit) and the action potentials are recorded at a more proximal site along the nerve trunk. In the antidromic method, the nerve trunk is stimulated at a proximal site and the response is recorded at a distal site (eg, from the digit). Antidromic digital studies tend to have higher amplitudes, because the recording electrodes are directly adjacent to the digital nerves. In orthodromic digital studies, the surface recording

---

Box 1
Motor nerve conduction study settings

Amplification: 2–5 mV/division

Sweep speed: 2–5 ms/division (occasionally increased when slowed conduction velocities)[5,6]

Filters: 2 Hz and 10 kHz

Table 1
Commonly performed motor nerve conduction studies

Nerve	Proximal Stimulation Sites	Distal Stimulation Site	Recorded Muscle
Bulbar			
Facial	—	Stylomastoid foramen	Nasalis
Spinal accessory	—	Posterior sternocleidomastoid	Trapezius
Upper extremity			
Median	Elbow at antecubital fossa	Wrist between flexor carpi radialis and palmaris longus tendons	Abductor pollicis brevis
Ulnar	Proximal to the medial epicondyle (and 2–4 cm distal to epicondyle)	Wrist medial to flexor carpi ulnaris tendon	Abductor digiti minimi or first dorsal interosseous
Radial	Spiral groove, axilla, and/or Erb point or axilla	Lateral epicondyle (elbow)	Extensor indicis proprius or extensor digitorum communis
Lower extremity			
Fibular	Knee medial to tendon of biceps femoris (and below fibular head)	Ankle lateral to the anterior tibialis tendon	Extensor digitorum brevis
Tibial	Knee at popliteal fossa	Ankle behind the medial malleolus	Abductor hallucis

Table 2
Less commonly performed motor nerve conduction studies

Nerve	Stimulation Sites	Recorded Muscle
Thorax		
Phrenic	Behind sternocleidomastoid at clavicle	Diaphragm over anterior chest
Upper extremity		
Axillary	Erb point	Deltoid
Suprascapular	Erb point	Supraspinatus/infraspinatus
Musculocutaneous	Anterior axillary fold and Erb point	Biceps brachii
Lower extremity		
Femoral	Inguinal ligament	Rectus femoris

Box 2
Sensory nerve conduction study settings

Amplification: 10 μV/division

Sweep speed: 1–2 ms/division

Filters: 20 Hz and 2 kHz

---

electrodes are separated from the nerve by subcutaneous tissue resulting in lower amplitudes. The stimulation site may need to be adjusted to achieve optimal stimulation when course of the nerve is variable.[3,4,9–12] Examples of the limb and digital type setups are shown in **Fig. 4**A–C. Examples of sensory NCS are shown in **Table 3**.

Mixed Nerve Conduction Studies

Mixed NCS refer to testing a nerve that contains sensory and motor axons. With this technique, a nerve with motor and sensory fibers is stimulated and the resulting action potentials are recorded from another site along the nerve. Common examples include midpalmar studies of the median and ulnar nerves and the medial plantar branch of the tibial nerve. Mixed studies are not a substitute for SNAPs when information about

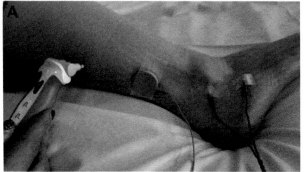
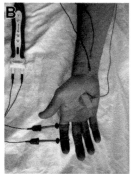
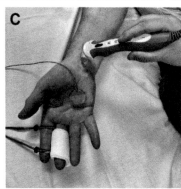

Fig. 4. Setups for the sural (A), median orthodromic (B), and median antidromic (C) sensory NCS. E0 (green) is between the stimulating and recording electrodes. The ring electrodes are the source of the stimuli in the orthodromic study and record the responses in the antidromic study. The gauze between digits II and III in the antidromic study prevents movement artifact from hand muscle contraction during stimulation.

Table 3
Sensory or mixed nerve conduction studies

Nerve	Stimulation Sites	Recording Sites
Bulbar		
Trigeminal (blink reflex)	Supraorbital notch	Ipsilateral/contralateral orbicularis oculi
Greater auricular	Lateral neck	Anterior to mastoid process
Upper extremity		
Orthodromic		
Median	2nd digit (or 1st/3rd/4th digits)	Elbow: antecubital fossa Wrist: between flexor carpi radialis and palmaris longus tendon
Ulnar	5th digit (or 4th digit)	Elbow: proximal to medial epicondyle Wrist: medial to flexor carpi ulnaris tendon
Antidromic		
Median	Wrist: between flexor carpi radialis and palmaris longus tendon Elbow: antecubital fossa	2nd digit (or 1st/3rd/4th digits)
Ulnar	Wrist: medial to the flexor carpi ulnaris tendon Elbow: proximal to the medial epicondyle	5th digit (or 4th digit)
Superficial radial	Lateral forearm	Wrist over the extensor pollicis longus tendon (or 1st digit)
Dorsal ulnar cutaneous	Medial forearm	Dorsal webspace between 4th and 5th digit
Medial antebrachial cutaneous	Antecubital fossa between biceps brachii tendon and medial epicondyle	Medial forearm
Lateral antebrachial cutaneous	Lateral to biceps brachii tendon	Lateral forearm
Mixed nerve		
Median	Palmar crease between 2nd and 3rd digits	Wrist: between flexor carpi radialis and palmaris longus tendons Elbow: antecubital fossa
Ulnar	Palmar crease between 4th and 5th digits	Wrist: medial to flexor carpi ulnaris

(continued on next page)

Table 3 (continued)		
Nerve	Stimulation Sites	Recording Sites
		tendon Elbow: proximal to medial epicondyle
Lower extremity		
Antidromic		
Sural	Lateral midcalf	Posterior to the lateral malleolus
Superficial fibular	Anterior lower leg posterior to insertion of peroneus longus	Ankle lateral to anterior tibialis tendon
Saphenous	Medial calf in groove between medial gastrocnemius and tibia	Ankle between the anterior tibialis tendon and medial malleolus
Mixed nerve		
Medial plantar	Medial to planter fascia at arch of the foot	Ankle behind medial malleolus
Lateral plantar	Lateral to plantar fascia at arch of the foot	Ankle behind medial malleolus

sensory function is needed. An example of the setup and action potentials from a mid-palmar NCS are shown in **Fig. 5**A,B.

NERVE CONDUCTION STUDY PARAMETERS

The features of the recorded CMAP and SNAP responses provide information about the integrity of the nerve axons and their myelination. CMAP responses also provide information on the functional integrity of the muscle and, using repetitive stimulation, the neuromuscular junction. Several parameters are quantified and compared with reference values. Abnormal values and morphologic features of the recorded waveforms can help to define the underlying pathologic process. Standard parameters

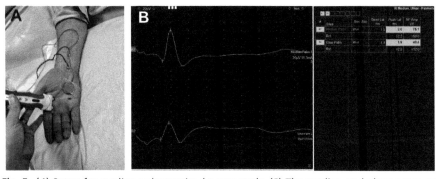

Fig. 5. (*A*) Setup for median palmar mixed nerve study. (*B*) The median and ulnar nerve action potentials resulting from midpalmar stimulation of the median (*top*) and ulnar (*bottom*) nerves.

evaluated include those related to conduction time along the nerve, such as distal latency (DL) and/or conduction velocity (CV), and the response amplitudes.

Conduction Time or Latency

Conduction time is traditionally measured (in milliseconds) as the latency between the time of stimulation to the appearance of the response. Latency is assessed over a fixed distance or is converted into a CV when variable nerve segment distances are tested. By convention, motor NCS latencies are measured to the onset of the negative component of the CMAP. Latencies recorded during sensory NCS have traditionally been measured to the negative peak of the SNAP, which is easier to identify than the onset latency. Modern instruments can average multiple responses allowing for more reliable determination of the onset latency. Onset or peak latency are equally valid; however, the values used should be compared with the appropriate reference values. Some sensory responses may have an initial positive component preceding the negative phase because of volume conducted activity at the E1 electrode. When an initial positive component is present, convention varies between whether the latency is measured from the initial deflection from the baseline or at the positive peak of that initial phase. Examples of motor and sensory latency determinations are shown in **Fig. 6**A, B.

In motor and sensory NCS, the DL is the conduction time between the distal (wrist or ankle) stimulation sites and the recorded response, and is a measure of the integrity of the myelin and axons in a distal segment of the nerve. It may be prolonged in disorders affecting distal segments of nerves, such as in a demyelinating median neuropathy at the wrist, ulnar neuropathy at the wrist, or distal polyneuropathy. The DL may be secondarily mildly prolonged when there is loss of large, fast conducting axons (see later).

Conduction Velocity

CV calculation normalizes differences in limb length and is calculated by dividing the length (in millimeters) of the nerve segment between two stimulation sites or a stimulation site and the E1 electrode (in millimeters) by the difference in conduction times (ie, difference in latencies of the recorded responses, in milliseconds) between those stimulation sites, using the following formula:

$$\text{Conduction velocity (m / s)} = \frac{\textit{distance between stimulation points}}{(\textit{proximal latency} - \textit{distal latency})}$$

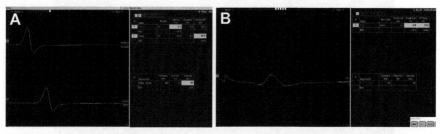

Fig. 6. Examples of standard methodology for marking response latency and amplitudes in motor (*A*) and sensory (*B*) NCS.

CV is most often calculated between the knee and ankle or elbow and wrist but can be calculated across any specific nerve segments, such as the ulnar nerve across elbow.

CV determination in the distal segment of a motor nerve is not an accurate measure of the conduction time along the nerves alone because of tapering of distal motor axons diameter, loss of myelination in the terminal branches, and the synaptic delay. Therefore, DL measurement using fixed distances and comparing with reference values using the same distances is more reliable. By contrast, CV calculation is a reliable measure of conduction in the distal segment of sensory nerves because delay of propagation across the neuromuscular junction is not a factor.

CV is a primary measure of the integrity of the myelin along a nerve. Focal or diffuse disorders that result in demyelination produce slowing of the CV. CV may be secondarily slowed in diseases characterized by loss of fast conducting axons.

Amplitude, Area, and Duration

The CMAP amplitude is a measure of the summation of muscle fiber action potentials. It directly reflects the number of functioning muscle fibers and indirectly reflects the number and function of motor axons and neuromuscular junctions. The CMAP amplitude is usually measured between the baseline and the waveform negative peak (see **Fig. 6**A, B). The CMAP area under the negative peak has similar significance as amplitude. In most normal nerves, the CMAP amplitudes and areas are similar at all stimulation sites, with only a mild decrease over distance. A reduction in the CMAP amplitude and area may occur in disorders that cause loss of motor axons (axonal neuropathies), muscle fibers (severe myopathies), or severe blocking at the neuromuscular junctions (eg, Lambert-Eaton myasthenic syndrome).

The duration of the CMAP negative phase is useful when assessing for multifocal or segmental demyelination within axons. When segmental demyelination occurs, axons conduct at variable rates and the recorded action potentials become more dispersed. When present, abnormal temporal dispersion between two stimulation sites helps to support acquired demyelination, such as may occur with inflammatory demyelination polyneuropathies. The CMAP duration may also be increased in disorders that impair conduction along muscle fibers, such as critical illness myopathy. **Fig. 7** illustrates area and duration determination.

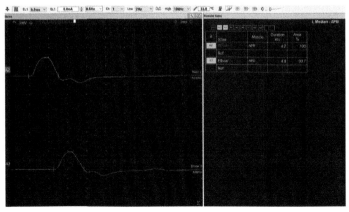

Fig. 7. CMAP duration and area measurements for a median motor NCS.

The SNAP amplitude reflects the number and timing of sensory axons; it is usually measured from baseline or initial positive peak to the negative peak. SNAP amplitudes are much lower than CMAP amplitudes and show much greater decline over longer nerve segment lengths than CMAPs as a result of phase cancellation between overlapping negative and positive phase components of the individual action potentials over longer distances.[13] **Fig. 8** shows normal ulnar SNAPs with wrist and elbow stimulation with a normal 33% decrease in amplitude between the two sites. SNAP amplitudes are reduced in disorders associated with loss of sensory axons.

Late Responses

Late responses refer to responses that occur after the CMAP and may be useful to assess more proximal segments of a nerve. There are several types of late responses.

F waves

During motor NCS, stimulation of the nerve at a distal site (eg, wrist or ankle) produces action potentials that propagate distally to the muscle, resulting in the direct CMAP, but also proximally, which reach the anterior horn cells. A small number of anterior horn cells may be depolarized by these action potentials and generate an orthodromic action potential that propagates back to the muscle. The resulting motor unit potentials were first recorded from foot muscles (F waves), although they are generated by the stimulation of any motor nerve (**Fig. 9**). F wave amplitudes are usually small (50–500 μV) and the configuration of each F waves varies during serial stimulation because of activation of different anterior horn cells.[14] F waves are most often interpreted by measuring their latencies (usually the earliest reproducible latency) during 8 to 12 distal serial supramaximal stimulations. F wave latencies may be prolonged in demyelinating processes that affect the nerve roots or proximal nerve segments, such as in Guillain-Barré syndrome, before CV slowing is seen on standard motor NCS. F waves may become undetectable in axon loss processes that result in CMAP amplitude reduction.[15,16]

A waves

Axon reflexes (or A waves) are late responses that may arise from axons that have developed collateral branches or are demyelinated. With distal nerve stimulation, action

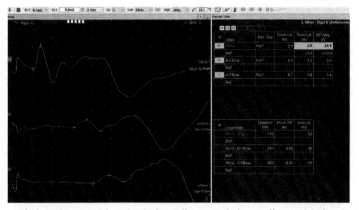

Fig. 8. Normal ulnar SNAPs with wrist, below elbow, and above elbow stimulus sites demonstrating a normal drop in amplitude between the wrist and below elbow traces. Each trace has been averaged 4 times.

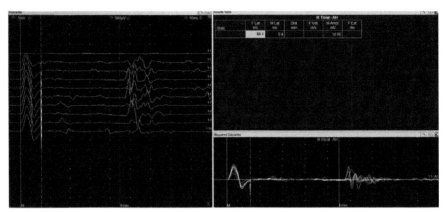

Fig. 9. Tibial F waves. Note the variation in configuration of each F wave because of different motor neurons being activated with sequential stimulation.

potentials propagating antidromically encounter the branch or ephaptically spread to a neighboring axon and propagate orthodromically back to muscle (**Fig. 10**). The constancy of latency and configuration of an axon reflex helps to distinguish A waves from F waves.[16] A waves are nonspecific and occur in any neurogenic process. Multiple A waves have also been reported as an early sign of Guillain-Barré syndrome.[17] They may occasionally be seen in normal individuals without apparent disease.

H reflex

The H reflex, named after Paul Hoffman who defined the characteristics of this response, is a late response that provides a quantifiable measure of the monosynaptic stretch reflex. It is observed during the stimulation of a mixed nerve by selective activation of sensory fibers that innervate the muscle spindles. This is accomplished by using a longer duration (1 millisecond), low-intensity stimulus. These sensory action potentials propagate proximally through the dorsal root ganglion and activate the monosynaptic reflex at the anterior horn cell, thereby producing an orthodromic motor response measured at the corresponding muscle. As stimulation levels are increased to maximal or supramaximal levels, the antidromic motor action potentials collide with orthodromic action potentials returning as part of the reflex arc, inhibiting the H reflex response (**Fig. 11**).[15]

The H reflex is most often used to evaluate the integrity of the S1 nerve roots and associated peripheral pathways in the sciatic nerve and sacral plexus with tibial (soleus recording) nerve stimulation. The median (flexor carpi radialis recording) H reflex may be used to assess the C7 root. H reflexes may be observed in other motor NCS in adults with upper motor neuron dysfunction.

PATTERNS OF NERVE CONDUCTION STUDY ABNORMALITIES

Various abnormalities on NCS can occur in neurogenic disorders associated with axonal loss or demyelination at any site along the lower motor neuron or peripheral sensory pathway, and in disorders directly involving the neuromuscular junctions or muscles.

Amplitude Reduction

Neurogenic disorders that result in axonal degeneration (eg, from compression, trauma, degeneration, ischemia) may lead to a decrease in CMAP amplitudes. The

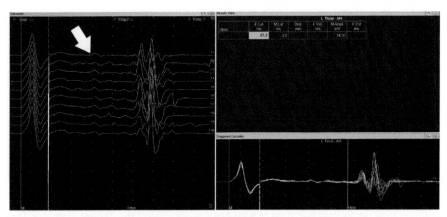

Fig. 10. Axon reflex or A wave (*arrow*) during a tibial motor NCS. The F waves follow each A wave. Note the identical A wave morphology but variable F wave configuration from trace to trace.

degree of amplitude reduction reflects the number of axons lost and the extent of rein-nervation. In disorders with loss of only few axons or when reinnervation has occurred, the amplitudes may not be significantly impacted or may remain normal. Reduction in CMAP amplitude may also occur in myopathies or severe neuromuscular junction disorders (**Table 4**).

Conditions that cause sensory axonal wallerian degeneration at or distal to the dorsal root ganglion result in a reduction or loss of SNAP amplitudes. In root compression, sensory axon degeneration occurs proximal to the dorsal root ganglion; therefore, the distal sensory NCS responses usually remain normal. In most axonal polyneuropathies, SNAPs become abnormal before CMAPs, and longer axons, such as to the distal legs and feet, are affected before those to the hands.[18]

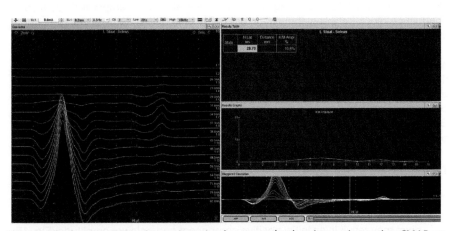

Fig. 11. Tibial motor NCS at increasing stimulus strengths showing an increasing CMAP on the *left* and later H reflex responses on the *right*. As stimulus strength is increased, the CMAP amplitude increases and the late response becomes an F wave in the last 5 traces. The late waveforms at lower stimulus levels are H reflexes.

Table 4		
NCS amplitudes in neuronopathies and radiculopathies		
	Motor NCS	**Sensory NCS**
Sensory neuronopathy	Normal	Low or absent
Motor neuronopathy	Low or absent (if severe)	Normal
Radiculopathy	Normal or low	Normal (rare exception: low superficial fibular in L5 radiculopathy)
Neuromuscular junction disorders	Normal (low if severe or presynaptic disease)	Normal
Myopathy	Normal or low	Normal

With axon loss that results in low amplitudes, mild CV slowing and/or slightly DL prolongation may be present because of a loss of a proportion of the largest diameter, fast conducting axons. The range of axon sizes in the large myelination population is such that axon loss only reduces CV to about 70% of the low limit of normal (eg, mid-30 m/s in upper limbs and about 30 m/s in the lower limbs).

Distal Latency Prolongation, Conduction Velocity Slowing, Conduction Block, and Abnormal Temporal Dispersion

Disorders that predominantly affect the myelin sheath produce prolonged DLs and slowed CV. Although these features are characteristic of demyelinating disorders, amplitudes may also become reduced in demyelinating diseases because of conduction block and secondary axonal injury.

When focal demyelination occurs to such a degree that the action potential is unable to propagate along the axon, a conduction block occurs. The CMAP amplitude is normal with stimulation distal to the block but low or absent with proximal stimulation. Inherited demyelinating neuropathies are usually associated with uniform demyelination along a nerve, resulting in similar waveform configurations along the nerve. Acquired disorders (eg, chronic inflammatory demyelinating polyneuropathy [CIDP] and acute inflammatory demyelinating polyneuropathy [AIDP]) produce segmental demyelination and nonuniform slowing, which produce abnormal temporal dispersion or conduction block between stimulation sites. Some acquired demyelinating neuropathies may affect motor more than sensory nerves, resulting in normal SNAPs.[18–21]

Pathology of the myelin and axons often coexist. Established NCS criteria for demyelination should be met to support a primarily demyelinating neuropathy, particularly in the context of low amplitudes. Additionally, needle EMG findings are helpful in distinguishing the presence and degree of axon involvement. Examples of NCS findings in predominantly axonal and demyelinating neuropathies are shown in **Figs. 12** and **13A, B**. Patterns of abnormality are summarized in **Table 5**. Examples of focal slowing and partial conduction block in NCS are shown in **Fig. 14A–C**.

TECHNICAL FACTORS IMPACTING NERVE CONDUCTION STUDIES

Many technical factors can affect reliable NCS results.

- Placement of the E1 recording electrode during motor NCS away from the motor point may result in an initial positive component and/or lower amplitude (**Fig. 15**).
- Excessive stimulus artifact during sensory NCS may affect the baseline and impact accurate determination of onset latency and amplitudes. Proper preparation of the skin at the electrode attachment sites, placement of the E0 electrode

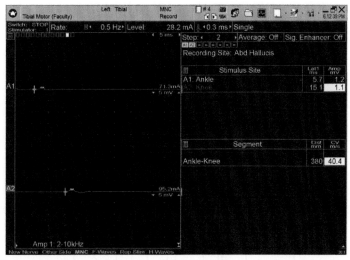

Fig. 12. Tibial motor NCS demonstrated low CMAP amplitudes in an axonal polyneuropathy. The conduction velocity is mildly slowed because of loss of a large number of large, fast conducting axons.

between the stimulating and recording electrodes, and slight rotation of the stimulator usually reduce stimulus artifact (**Fig. 16**).

- Placement of the recording electrodes farther from a sensory nerve may result in a reduction in the SNAP amplitude.
- During sensory NCS, distortion of the SNAP may occur because of volume conduction of CMAPs from nearby muscles. This often occurs during antidromic ulnar sensory studies. Moving the E1 electrode 1 to 2 cm distally on the digit often reduces the motor artifact (**Fig. 17**).
- Stimulator sliding away from the nerve may result in depolarization of fewer axons and low or absent responses.

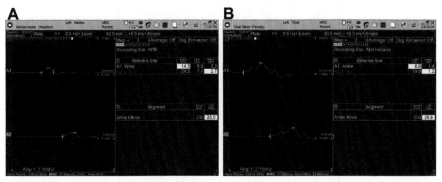

Fig. 13. (*A*) Median motor NCS results from a patient with Charcot-Marie-Tooth type 1 are shown. Note the similar configurations of the distal and proximal CMAPs, the prolonged distal latency, and the very slow CV. (*B*) Tibial motor NCS results from a patient with chronic inflammatory demyelinating neuropathy. Note the change in configuration between distal and proximal stimulation sites and the slow CV and prolonged distal latency.

Table 5
NCS findings in axonal and demyelinating neuropathies

	Sensory		Motor			
	Distal Latency	Amplitude	Distal Latency	Amplitude	Conduction Velocity	F Waves
Axonal						
Mild	NL	Low (if sensory)	NL	NL	NL or mildly slowed	NL or mildly prolonged
Severe	NL or mildly prolonged	Low or absent	NL or mildly prolonged	Low or absent	Mildly slowed	Absent
Demyelinating						
Uniform	Prolonged	NL (low if severe)	Prolonged	NL	Slowed	Prolonged
Segmental	NL or prolonged (if distal segments involved)	NL (low if severe)	NL or prolonged (if distal segments involved)	Low (conduction block or abnormal dispersion)	Slowed	Prolonged

Abbreviation: NL, normal.

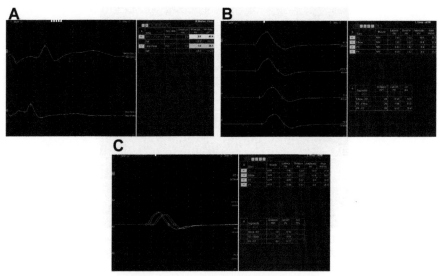

Fig. 14. (A) Prolongation of the mixed nerve action potential in a median palmar mixed study in contrast to normal latency in the ulnar segment of the same length. (B) The series of CMAPs from an ulnar motor NCS illustrate focal prolongation of latency between stimulus sites 2 cm apart along the nerve in the elbow region. Note the larger latency increase at the site of maximum abnormality. (C) Drop in the ulnar CMAP amplitude at the lesion site in the elbow segment as the stimulator is moved 2 cm proximally between each trace, in a technique referred to as inching. Conduction block in some axons accounts for the amplitude decrease.

- Overstimulation may result in current spread to adjacent nerves with recruitment of those axons, producing a falsely higher response.
- Cool limb temperature significantly impacts DLs and CVs. Foot and hand temperatures should be measured before beginning an NCS and monitored

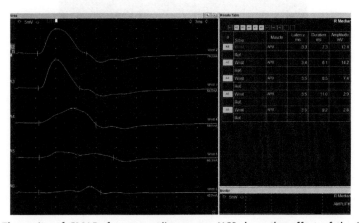

Fig. 15. The series of CMAPs from a median motor NCS show the effect of the E1 being located off the optimal recording site over the thenar muscles. Note the lower amplitudes and altered configurations compared with the top trace.

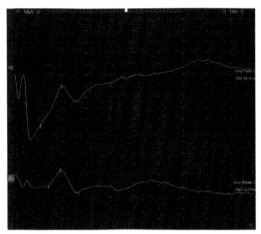

Fig. 16. Distortion of the onset of the ulnar SNAP because of excessive stimulus artifact (*top*). Rotation of the stimulator often reduces the stimulus artifact (*bottom*).

throughout the study. The minimum temperature for reliable NCS is 32.5°C in the hands and 30°C in the feet.[22] Latency increases approximately 0.15 milliseconds and CV decreases by about 2.5 m/s for each degree Centigrade less than the lower temperature limits. Amplitude and duration increase with cool limb temperature, particularly in SNAPs.[23,24] Cool limbs should be warmed (eg, with warming blankets or gel packs or immersion of a limb in warm water) for at least 5 minutes before testing (**Fig. 18A–C**).

- Errors in result interpretation can occur if nonstandardized reference or normative values are used. The 2016 normative NCS data project of the American Association of Neuromuscular & Electrodiagnostic Medicine recommended values for most standard NCS based on an extensive literature review.[25]

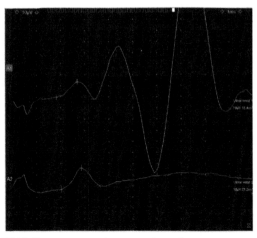

Fig. 17. This ulnar SNAP illustrates a volume conducted motor response from ulnar hand muscles altering the SNAP in the top trace. The lower trace shows the effect of moving E1 1 cm distal in the proximal phalanx.

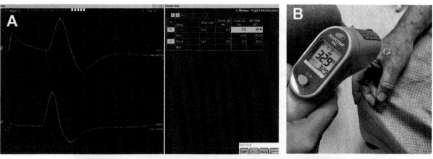

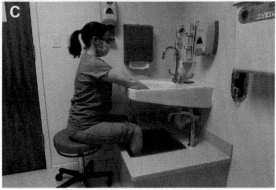

Fig. 18. (*A*) The effect of cool temperature on median SNAPs. The upper trace was recorded when the temperature in the digit was 28°C. The lower trace shows reduction in latency after the hand had been warmed by immersion in 40°C water for 5 minutes. (*B*) Determination of hand temperature by a handheld infrared thermometer is shown. (*C*) Warming hands and feet in a sink and foot tub.

SUMMARY

NCS are a key component of the electrophysiologic evaluation of the peripheral nerve system, and provide important information about the integrity of the large, myelinated axons, neuromuscular junctions, and muscle. Attention to details of test performance, use of well-established normative values, and knowledge of the patterns of abnormality produced by disorders that affect neuronal, axonal, and myelin sheath function are fundamental for proper interpretation of results.

CLINICS CARE POINTS

- NCS is valuable for evaluating the integrity of large, myelinated motor and sensory axons, as well as the neuromuscular junctions and the muscles. Small myelinated and unmyelinated axons are not assessed by standard NCS.
- NCS can test motor, sensory and mixed nerves, and can be utilized to study upper and lower extremities as well as bulbar responses.
- NCS parameters include conduction time or latency, amplitude, conduction velocity, area and duration. These parameters can be applied to both the CMAP and SNAP responses.
- Late responses refer to responses that occur after the CMAP and may be useful to assess more proximal segments of a nerve, and include F waves, A waves and the H reflex.

- Neurogenic disorders that result in axonal degeneration (such as from compression, trauma, degeneration, ischemia, etc.), may lead to a decrease in CMAP and SNAP amplitudes and mild slowing of conduction velocity.
- Disorders that predominantly affect the myelin sheath produce prolonged distal latencies and very slowed conduction velocities.
- Many technical factors can affect reliable NCS results, including incorrect electrode placement, artifact, cold temperature, as well as interpretation errors.

DISCLOSURE

Textbook author, Prahlow, ND, Kincaid, JC. Rehabilitation Medicine Quick Reference, Neuromuscular. RM, Buschbacher, Editor. New York: Demos Medical Publishing; 2014.

REFERENCES

1. Misulis K. Basic electronics for clinical neurophysiology. J Clin Neurophysiol 1989;6(1):41–71.
2. Instrumentation. In: Dumitru D, Amato A, Zwarts, editors. Electrodiagnostic medicine. 2nd edition. Philadelphia: Hanley & Belfus; 2002. p. 69–114.
3. Kincaid J, Brashear A, Markand O. The influence of the reference electrode on CMAP configuration. Muscle & Nerve 1993;16(4):392–6.
4. Nandedkar S, Barkhaus P. Contribution of the reference electrode to the compound muscle action potential. Muscle & Nerve 2007;36:87–92.
5. Hodes R, Larrabee M, German W. The human electromyogram in response to nerve stimulation and the conduction velocity of motor nerves. Arch Neurol Psychiatry 1948;60:340–65.
6. Jones L, Watson J. Motor nerve conductions: compound muscle action potentials. In: Rubin D, Daube J, editors. Clinical neurophysiology. 4th edition. New York: Oxford University Press; 2016. p. 257–91.
7. Preston D, Shapiro B. Electromyography and neuromuscular disorders. 4th edition. Philadelphia Elsevier; 2021. p. 107–33.
8. Kumbhare D, Robinson L, Buschbacher R. Bushbacher's manual of nerve conduction studies. 3rd edition. New York: Demos Medical; 2016.
9. Buchthal F, Rosenfalck A. Evoked action potentials and conduction velocities in human sensory nerves. Brain Res 1966;3:1–122.
10. Wilbourn AJ. Sensory conduction studies. J Clin Neurophysiol 1994;11:584–601.
11. Sorenson E. Sensory nerve action potentials. In: Rubin D, Dauble J, editors. Clinical neurophysiology. 4th edition. New York: Oxford University Press; 2016. p. 292–311.
12. Cohn T, Wertsch J, Pasupuleti D. Nerve conduction studies: orthodromic vs antidromic latencies. Arch Phys Med Rehabil 1990;71:579–82.
13. Kincaid J, Minnick K, Pappas S. A model of the differing change in motor and sensory action over distance. Muscle & Nerve 1988;11:318–23.
14. Fisher MA, Hoffen B, Hultman C. Normative F-wave values and the number of recorded F-waves. Muscle & Nerve 1994;17:1185–9.
15. Fisher MA. AANEM Minimonograph #13: H reflexes and F-waves: physiology and clinical indications. Muscle & Nerve 1992;15:1223–33.
16. The F wave and the A wave, Kimura J. Electrodiagnosis in diseases of the nerve and muscle. 4th edition. New York: Oxford; 2013. p. 149–73.

17. Kornhuber ME, Bischoff H, Mentrup H, et al. Multiple A waves in Guillain-Barré syndrome. Muscle & Nerve 1999;22:394–9.
18. The H. T and Masseter and Silent Period, . Kimura J. Electrodiagnosis in diseases of the nerve and muscle. 4th edition. New York: Oxford; 2013. p. 208–22.
19. Albers J. Clinical neurophysiology of generalized polyneuropathy. J Clin Neurophysiol 1993;10:149–66.
20. Dyck P, Lamber E, Mulder D. Charcot Marie Toot disease: nerve conduction and clinical studies in a large kindred. Neurology 1963;13(11):1–11.
21. Lewis R. Sumner A. The electrodiagnostic distinction between chronic familial and acquired demyelinating neuropathies. Neurology 2000;23(10):1472–87.
22. American Association of Neuromuscular and Electrodiagnostic Medicine. Reporting the results of needle EMG and nerve conduction studies: an educational report. Muscle Nerve 2014;1–6. AANEM Practice Topic.
23. Technical Issues and Potential Complications of Nerve Conduction Studies. In: Rubin D, Daube J, editors. Clinical neurophysiology. 4th edition. New York: Oxford University Press; 2016. p. 382–3.
24. Deny EH. AANEM minimonography #14: The influence of temperature in clinical neurophysiology. Muscle & Nerve 1991;14:795–811.
25. Chen S, Andary M, Buschbacher R, et al. Electrodiagnostic reference values for upper and lower limb nerve conduction studies in adults. Muscle & Nerve 2016; 54:371–7.

Needle Electromyography Waveforms During Needle Electromyography

Devon I. Rubin, MD

KEYWORDS

- Needle electromyography • Waveforms • Fibrillation potentials
- Motor unit potentials • Spontaneous activity

KEY POINTS

- Needle electromyography (EMG) waveforms are identified by their firing patterns.
- Spontaneous waveforms may indicate abnormalities within the muscle fibers or axons; most are nonspecific and can be seen in many neuromuscular disorders.
- Analysis of voluntary motor unit potentials helps to determine the type of neuromuscular disorder and the chronicity and severity of the disorder.

INTRODUCTION

Needle electromyography (EMG) records the electrical signals generated from muscle fibers within a muscle. These signals provide information regarding the function of motor units, neuromuscular junctions, and muscle fibers. In neuromuscular diseases, abnormal spontaneously generated signals or alterations in the voluntary motor unit potentials (MUPs) may occur. The presence and characteristics of these signals can be extrapolated to determine the presence, type, chronicity, and severity of disease.

Different EMG potentials may have identical morphologies; therefore, distinguishing the different waveforms requires recognition of their firing patterns, which may be regular, irregular, or semirhythmic (**Fig. 1**). During MUP assessment, 20 to 30 different MUPs are measured, and the average size and morphology of the MUPs are determined, either by semiquantitative measurement or formal quantitative methods. Several quantitative measures may be used during low to strong contraction, each with benefits and limitations.[1–6]

Many publications review the EMG waveforms, and standards for quantification of EMG waveforms have been recently published.[7–9] This article reviews the significance of EMG waveforms through clinical problems that may present to the EMG laboratory.

The author has no financial disclosures relevant to this article.
Department of Neurology, Mayo Clinic, 4500 San Pablo Road, Jacksonville, FL 32224, USA
E-mail address: Rubin.devon@mayo.edu

Neurol Clin 39 (2021) 919–938
https://doi.org/10.1016/j.ncl.2021.06.003
0733-8619/21/© 2021 Elsevier Inc. All rights reserved.

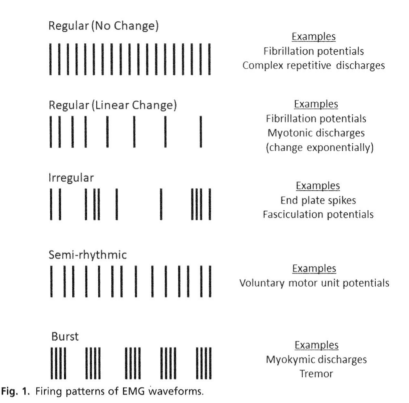

Fig. 1. Firing patterns of EMG waveforms.

CASE 1. INCREASED INSERTION ACTIVITY AND ENDPLATE ACTIVITY

A 38-year-old man presented with diffuse muscle aching. NCS were normal. Needle examination demonstrated increased insertional activity with brief runs of positive waves following cessation of needle movement. No fibrillation potentials or other abnormal spontaneous discharges were recorded, and MUPs were normal. The interpretation was nonspecific increased insertional activity, which could be a benign variant but can also be seen in subtle myotonic myopathies.

Insertion Activity

As the needle moves though a resting muscle, it irritates individual muscle fibers and generates muscle fiber action potentials. These induced action potentials are referred to as insertion activity.[10] Bursts of insertion activity may be composed of few spikes or many spikes, depending on the length of needle movement.[11] (**Fig. 2**) Once the needle movement has ceased, the recorded spikes should also cease.[12] Insertion activity can be increased or decreased in different diseases.

Increased insertion activity

Electrical activity that persists following cessation of needle movement is increased insertional activity[13] (see **Fig. 2**). Increased insertion activity may occur as a benign variant as irregular, occasional spikes that persist for a variable time following cessation of needle movement (termed "snap, crackle, pop"). When present, this is typically seen diffusely and is more common in younger men.[14] A second variant is brief, non-sustained runs of positive waves.[15] In rare cases, patients' brief runs of positive waves

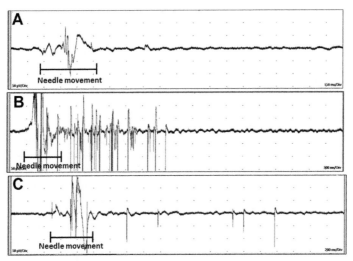

Fig. 2. Examples of insertion activity. (*A*) Normal. (*B*) Increased. (*C*) Snap, crackle, pop.

that resemble fragments of myotonic discharges have been found in myotonia congenita or myotonic dystrophy type 2.[16–18] Increased insertion activity more often occurs early in fiber denervation (eg, subacute radiculopathy), even before distinct fibrillation potentials develop.[19,20]

Decreased insertion activity
Decreased insertion activity occurs with severe muscle atrophy, replacement of muscle tissue by fat or connective tissue (such as end-stage myopathies or neurogenic disorders), or in electrically silent muscles (eg, during an attack of periodic paralysis or a contracture in metabolic myopathies). In these instances, movement of the needle electrode through the muscle will not result in a burst of spikes.

Endplate Activity

Two types of waveforms are recorded at the endplate region – endplate spikes and endplate noise. Endplate noise represents the miniature endplate potentials resulting from the spontaneous release of individual quanta of acetylcholine from the presynaptic nerve ending.[21] When the needle electrode irritates a terminal nerve branch, release of multiple quanta of acetylcholine from its nerve ending occurs, resulting in generation of an action potential called an endplate spike.[22] (**Fig. 3**) Endplate spikes fire in an irregular pattern. Endplate activity is a normal finding.

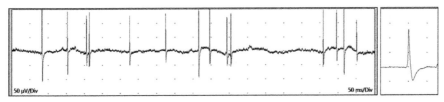

Fig. 3. Endplate spikes.

CASE 2. FIBRILLATION POTENTIALS AND NORMAL VOLUNTARY MOTOR UNIT POTENTIALS

Needle EMG of a 56-year old man referred evaluation of a right lumber radiculopathy demonstrated 2+ fibrillation potentials in the right peroneus longus, posterior tibialis, tensor fascia lata, and L5 paraspinal muscles. MUPs were normal in all muscles. The interpretation was subacute, active right L5 radiculopathy.

Fibrillation Potentials

Fibrillation potentials are the spontaneously firing action potentials of single muscle fibers when the fibers have been denervated.[13] The precise mechanism of generation of fibrillation potentials is not known but is thought to be the result of reduced threshold for action potential generation and denervation hypersensitivity at the endplate zone - all resulting in a spontaneous, regularly firing, recurring action potential.[23–25] Fibrillation potentials usually take 14 to 21 days to develop following an acute nerve injury, but the timing partially depends on the distance of the muscle from the site of nerve injury. Muscles closer to the site of injury demonstrate fibrillation potentials earlier than more distant muscles.[26] Fibrillation potentials fire in a regular pattern and may have a spike form or positive wave form (positive sharp waves)[27,28] (**Fig. 4**).

The significance of fibrillation potentials depends on the clinical context in which they are recorded and the temporal course of the patient's symptoms. Fibrillation potentials may occur from denervation in a variety of neurogenic disorders or because of destruction of the muscle fiber in many myopathies[23,25] (**Table 1**).

Fibrillation potentials in radiculopathies

When axons at the root level undergo Wallerian degeneration, muscle fibers supplied by the damaged axons lose their innervation, resulting in fibrillation potentials. Fibrillation potentials develop earlier in muscles that are in closer proximity to the site of injury (eg, parapinals, gluteus medius) than distant muscles (eg, peroneus longus). The density of fibrillation potentials reflects the number of fibers denervated and

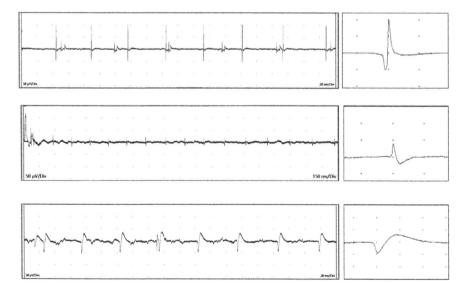

Fig. 4. Examples of 3 morphologies of fibrillation potentials – triphasic (*top*), biphasic, initially negative (*middle*), and positive wave (*bottom*).

Type of Disorder	Examples
Anterior horn cell diseases	Amyotrophic lateral sclerosis (ALS), spinal muscular atrophy, acute viral
Polyradiculopathies (axonal)	
Radiculopathies	Active or old with incomplete reinnervation
Plexopathies	
Polyneuropathies (axonal)	
Mononeuropathies	More severe with motor involvement
Neuromuscular junction disorders	Severe (eg, botulism)
Myopathies	Inflammatory Necrotizing Infiltrative (eg, amyloid) Muscular dystrophies Medications (eg, statins) Metabolic (eg, acid maltase deficiency) Congenital (eg, myotubular) Infectious (eg, viral)

Table 1
Disorders associated with fibrillation potentials

severity (**Fig. 5**). When the fibers become reinnervated, fibrillation potentials disappear. However, fibrillation potentials may persist in distal limb muscles, even in the context of a resolving or recovering radiculopathy. Furthermore, in severe root injuries, complete reinnervation may never fully occur, and some fibrillation potentials may persist indefinitely. Therefore, while the presence of fibrillation potentials often implies

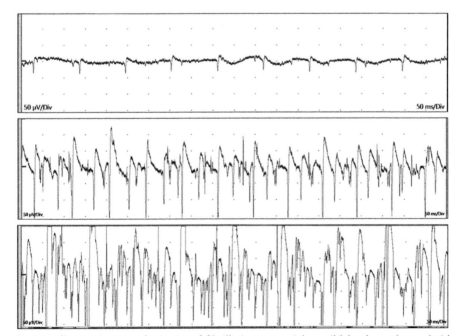

Fig. 5. Different degrees of severity of fibrillation potentials – mild (*top*), moderate (*middle*), and severe (*bottom*).

an active radiculopathy, they may be present as the residua of an old process. Therefore, the distribution of fibrillation potentials and the time course of the patient's symptoms must be considered.

Fibrillation potentials in other neurogenic disorders

In compressive mononeuropathies (eg, carpal tunnel syndrome) in which sensory axons are more susceptible to injury than motor fibers, the presence of fibrillation potentials often suggests a more severe process.[29] Fibrillation potentials are a characteristic, defining feature in motor neuron diseases such as ALS; however, they may not be present early in the course of the disease if reinnervation is keeping up with motor neuron degeneration. Similarly, in chronic or very slowly progressive axonal neuropathies, fibrillation potentials may be sparse or minimal until the nerves have lost their capability to reinnervate a muscle.

Fibrillation potentials in myopathies

Fibrillation potentials occur in myopathies characterized pathologically by muscle fiber necrosis, fiber splitting, infiltrative myopathies, and those associated with the formation of vacuoles that separate portions of a fiber.[25,30]

Normal Voluntary Motor Unit Potentials

Voluntary MUPs represent the action potentials of a group of near synchronous firing muscle fibers in the region of the recording electrode, innervated by the same anterior horn cell and axon. The features of a MUP can be extrapolated to assess the size and integrity of its motor unit.

Several MUP parameters are assessed for each MUP, each reflecting a physiologic measure of motor unit activation or morphology. Each of these parameters may be altered in diseases, depending on the pathology, temporal course, and severity.

Recruitment

The number of active motor units can be indirectly estimated during needle EMG by assessing MUP recruitment. MUP recruitment is defined by the relationship between the number of MUPs present with a specific level of contraction and the firing rates of individual MUPs.[31,32] It can be assessed by determining the recruitment frequency (the firing rate of the initially firing MUP when the second MUP is activated) or the recruitment ratio (the ratio of the fastest firing rate of any MUP near the needle electrode and the number of nearby MUPs that are firing). Recruitment may be altered in diseases, resulting in loss of functioning motor units (**Fig. 6**). With loss of anterior horn cells or axons or block of conduction along axons, central activation is increased, causing the remaining MUPs to fire at higher frequencies to attempt to generate a sustained tetanic contraction, yet fewer MUPs are able to discharge (reduced recruitment).[33] Reduced recruitment may be the only abnormality in an acute neurogenic disorder and may occur immediately after a nerve injury, before fibrillation potentials or MUP configuration changes develop.

Stability

MUP stability refers to the moment-to-moment change in the MUP configuration as it repeatedly fires during sustained contraction. Stability is a marker of the adequacy of neuromuscular transmission. Normal motor units have a stable appearance (ie, the MUP looks and sounds the same each time it fires). Impaired neuromuscular transmission results in unstable or varying MUP.[34] Unstable MUPs are characteristic of neuromuscular junction disorders but are more commonly seen in neurogenic disorders when early or ongoing reinnervation is occurring.

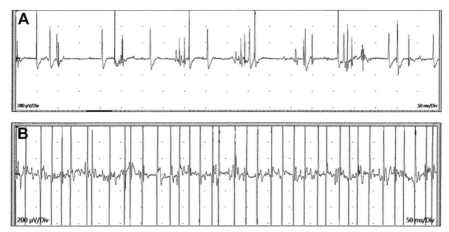

Fig. 6. MUP recruitment examples. (*A*) Normal recruitment with 4 different motor unit potentials firing at low rates. (*B*) Reduced recruitment with 1 MUP firing at approximately 40 Hz.

Phases/Turns

The timing of firing of each of the fibers composing an MUP varies slightly because of variations in the length and myelination of terminal nerves, variation in the conduction time along muscle fibers, and distance of muscle fibers to the recording electrode. Because conduction along the nerve and muscle fiber is similar for most fibers, most normal MUPs are triphasic. With reinnervation of muscle fibers or loss of fibers in a motor unit (in myopathies), there is more variability in the timing of recording the muscle fibers, and MUPs become more polyphasic (**Fig. 7**). A phase is defined as the number of baseline crossings plus one, and most MUPs have less than 4 phases.[35] An MUP that has 5 or more phases is considered polyphasic. In reinnervating neurogenic disorders, polyphasic MUPs begin to develop approximately 4 weeks after an acute nerve injury.[36] Turns are defined by a change in direction of a spike that does not cross the baseline and have similar significance as phases.

Duration, amplitude, area

The size of any MUP can be defined by several parameters, all of which reflect the number of fibers of the motor unit within the recording area, the distribution of fibers of a motor unit, and the timing of firing of the fibers within a motor unit. Common parameters include duration and amplitude. Other parameters such as area, thickness, and size index have been shown to be more reliable parameters to distinguish neurogenic and myopathic disorders from normal but have less defined reference values.[35,37–39] In neurogenic disorders associated with reinnervation, all the size parameters increase, usually beginning approximately 1 month after injury and continuing for months or years as reinnervation continues. In myopathic disorders, the size parameters decrease.

CASE 3. FASCICULATION POTENTIALS AND LONG DURATION, UNSTABLE MOTOR UNIT POTENTIALS WITH REDUCED RECRUITMENT

A 70-year-old woman was referred for 6 months of hand weakness and atrophy. Her NCS demonstrated low median and ulnar CMAP amplitudes with normal sensory responses. Needle EMG demonstrates fibrillation potentials, fasciculation potentials,

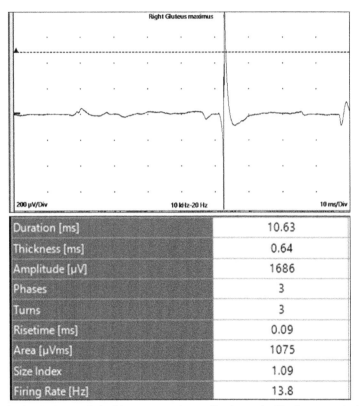

Duration [ms]	10.63
Thickness [ms]	0.64
Amplitude [μV]	1686
Phases	3
Turns	3
Risetime [ms]	0.09
Area [μVms]	1075
Size Index	1.09
Firing Rate [Hz]	13.8

Fig. 7. A single MUP recorded with a concentric needle electrode. The bottom window demonstrates the values of each measured parameter of that MUP.

and long duration, unstable, polyphasic MUPs with reduced recruitment in multiple arm, leg, and thoracic muscles. The interpretation was progressive diffuse neurogenic disorder, consistent with motor neuron disease.

Fasciculation Potentials

Fasciculation potentials represent the action potentials of spontaneous firing motor units. The morphologies reflect the size of its underlying motor unit. When present in chronic neurogenic disorders, fasciculation potentials are often large and polyphasic. Fasciculations fire in an irregular firing pattern[7,9] (**Fig. 8**). They are nonspecific and seen in individuals without neuromuscular diseases but are frequent in those with neurogenic disorders (**Table 2**). Although they are part of the diagnostic criteria for amyotrophic lateral sclerosis as a marker of lower motor neuron involvement, in the absence of neurogenic MUP changes or fibrillation potentials, fasciculation potentials alone are not diagnostic of a lower motor neuron disorder.[40]

Reduced Recruitment, Unstable, Long Duration Motor Unit Potentials

Reduced recruitment in neurogenic disorders

Reduced recruitment is a marker of loss of motor units and characteristic of a neurogenic disorder. Reduced recruitment alone does not reflect chronicity of a process, as it can occur acutely or be present indefinitely, even decades following a nerve injury.[41]

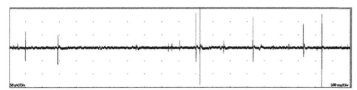

Fig. 8. Fasciculation potentials recorded during needle EMG. The display sweep is 500 milliseconds per division.

Motor unit potential instability and increased size in neurogenic disorders

In chronic or evolving neurogenic disorders, fibers that have lost their innervation are reinnervated through collateral sprouting, resulting in long-duration, high-amplitude MUPs.[36,42] (**Fig. 9**) With early or ongoing reinnervation, neuromuscular transmission is impaired in the newly reinnervated fibers, which is seen as unstable MUPs.[43] Thus, unstable MUPs with increased duration indicate a neurogenic process with ongoing reinnervation. This pattern begins weeks following an acute nerve injury and can be seen in chronic disorders associated with ongoing loss of motor units with ongoing reinnervation.

CASE 4. MYOTONIC DISCHARGES AND SHORT DURATION, POLYPHASIC MOTOR UNIT POTENTIALS WITH RAPID (EARLY) RECRUITMENT

A 32-year-old woman was referred for muscle stiffness. Her examination demonstrated mild distal arm and leg weakness. NCS were normal. Needle EMG demonstrated myotonic discharges in most muscles, fibrillation potentials in distal muscles, and short-duration, low-amplitude, polyphasic MUPs with rapid recruitment in distal more than proximal muscles. The interpretation was myopathy with myotonic discharges, possible myotonic dystrophy type 1.

Myotonic Discharges

Myotonic discharges are the action potentials of single muscle fibers that fire spontaneously or are induced by needle movement or muscle contraction.[44] They develop in disorders associated with impaired muscle fiber sodium or chloride channels, which result in abnormal afterdepolarization of the action potential and a repetitive firing action potential.[45,46] Myotonic discharges have a characteristic firing pattern of exponentially increasing and decreasing firing rates (**Fig. 10**). The amplitude of each spike within the discharges may increase and decrease. The discharges can be brief

Table 2		
Disorders associated with fasciculation potentials		
Type of Disorder	**Examples**	
No disorder	Benign fasciculation syndrome	
Neurogenic disorders	Anterior horn cell diseases Peripheral neuropathies Radiculopathies	
Peripheral nerve hyperexcitable disorders	Cramp fasciculation syndrome Isaac syndrome	
Medications	Pyridostigmine	
Metabolic disorders	Hyperthyroidism	

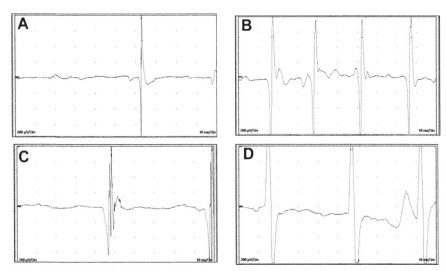

Fig. 9. Changes in MUPs with time following an acute neurogenic process. (*A*) Normal MUP. (*B*) Reduced recruitment with normal morphology. (*C*) Mildly increased phases. (*D*) Long duration, high amplitude, triphasic.

or long, and the firing rates of the spikes range from 10 to 100 Hz.[47] When recorded diffusely or in multiple muscles, myotonic discharges indicate myotonic myopathies or muscle channelopathies (**Table 3**). However, isolated myotonic discharges may be recorded in a few muscles in other myopathies, including necrotizing and inflammatory myopathies.[48,49]

Rapid (Early) Recruitment

In myopathies associated with destruction and/or loss of function of muscle fibers, less force is generated from the muscle when the motor unit fires. To compensate for this, more anterior horn cells fire to activate more muscle fibers to generate a necessary force. With low effort, more motor units are recruited than normal, termed rapid or early recruitment.[50] Rapid recruitment is mostly determined subjectively based on the expected number of muscle fibers relative to the amount of effort given by the patient, and is usually seen as greater than 5 MUPs with normal firing rates activated with minimal contraction. Rapid recruitment is characteristic of myopathies, although not all myopathies demonstrate this pattern.

Short-Duration, Polyphasic Motor Unit Potentials

In many myopathies, fewer muscle fiber action potentials are present in the recording area, producing a short-duration, low-amplitude MUP. Furthermore, because the remaining action potentials may fire less synchronously, the MUP may be polyphasic.[51–53] (**Fig. 11**) These features are characteristic of myopathies associated with fiber necrosis, fiber splitting, or other mechanisms that destroy or break down individual muscle fibers (**Table 4**). Myopathies that are not associated with muscle fiber destruction or loss or that involve type 2 muscle fibers, (eg, corticosteroid, endocrine, and some metabolic or congenital myopathies) may not produce changes in the MUP morphology. Furthermore, in chronic myopathies with ongoing reinnervation or regeneration of fibers, the duration and amplitude of the MUP may remain in the normal range (or even be long).

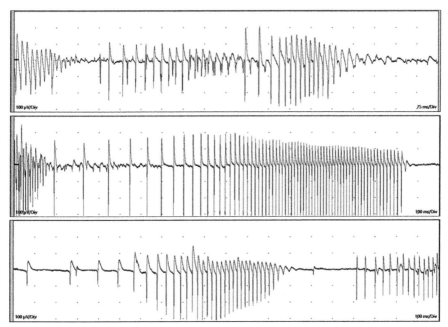

Fig. 10. Examples of myotonic discharges.

Low-amplitude, short-duration, polyphasic MUPs (with instability and reduced recruitment) also occur as nascent MUPs in newly formed MUPs from early reinnervation following severe nerve injury (**Fig. 12**).

CASE 5. UNSTABLE MOTOR UNIT POTENTIALS

A 60-year woman was referred for left eyelid ptosis and diplopia. Routine NCS and repetitive nerve stimulation were normal. Needle examination demonstrated unstable MUPs of normal duration and amplitude and normal recruitment in the frontalis. The findings are consistent with a disorder of neuromuscular transmission, such as myasthenia gravis.

Table 3
Disorders with myotonic discharges

Type of Disorder	Examples
Myotonic dystrophies	Myotonic dystrophy type 1 and type 2
Muscle channelopathies	Myotonia congenita
	Paramyotonia congenita Hyperkalemic periodic paralysis
Metabolic myopathies	Acid maltase deficiency
Congenital myopathies	Centronuclear, caveolin-3 mutation, myofibrillar
Necrotizing myopathies	
Inflammatory myopathies	
Infiltrative myopathies	Amyloidosis
Medications	Statins
Chronic neurogenic disorders	Axonal polyneuropathy

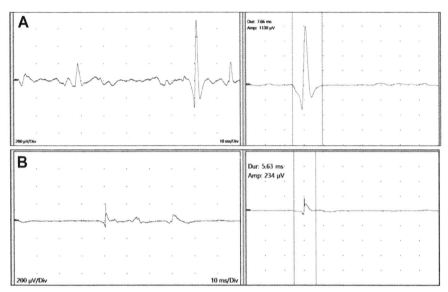

Fig. 11. Comparison of a normal MUP (*A*) and short-duration, low-amplitude MUP in a myopathy (*B*).

When neuromuscular transmission is impaired, endplate potentials are not large enough to reach the threshold for action potential generation, and an action potential is blocked from being generated along that fiber. As a result, variable numbers of muscle fiber action potentials are summated with each discharge of the motor unit, and the MUP morphology changes each time it fires, producing an unstable MUP[54] (**Fig. 13**). Unstable MUPs are characteristic of neuromuscular junction diseases, such as myasthenia gravis or Lambert Eaton myasthenic syndrome, but are not specific and commonly occur in neurogenic disorders in which reinnervation and motor unit remodeling is occurring (**Table 5**).

Table 4
Disorders associated with short duration, low amplitude motor unit potentials

Type of Disease	Examples
Myopathies	Muscular dystrophies
	Inflammatory
	Necrotizing
	Infiltrative
	Congenital
	Endocrine
	Medications (not corticosteroids)
Neuromuscular junction disorders	Severe myasthenia gravis
	Lambert-Eaton myasthenic syndrome
	Botulism
Neurogenic disorders	Early reinnervation after severe injury (nascent MUP)
No disease	Infants and young pediatric patients
	(MUPs are normally small)

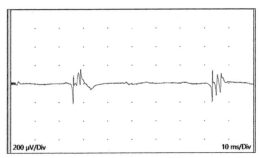

Fig. 12. Nascent (low amplitude, short duration, unstable, polyphasic with reduced recruitment) MUP following severe nerve injury.

CASE 6. COMPLEX REPETITIVE DISCHARGES AND LONG DURATION, HIGH-AMPLITUDE MOTOR UNIT POTENTIALS

A 75-year-old man was referred for a 6-week history of right back and buttock pain. NCS demonstrated a low right fibular motor compound muscle action potential amplitude with a normal tibial motor and sural amplitude. Needle examination demonstrated no fibrillation potentials but long-duration, triphasic MUPs in the right anterior tibialis, peroneus longus, and tensor fascia lata. Complex repetitive discharges (CRDs) were recorded in the tensor fascia lata. Interpretations were old, inactive right L5 radiculopathy.

Complex Repetitive Discharges

CRDs are spontaneous discharges composed of groups of time-locked muscle fiber action potentials that recur in a regular firing pattern. Each repeating group may be

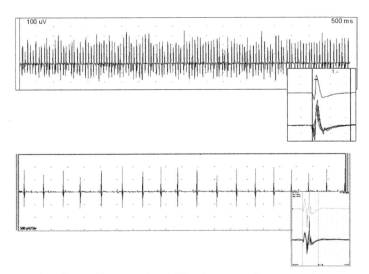

Fig. 13. Examples of unstable or varying MUPs, demonstrating moment-to-moment amplitude change. The top example is at a sweep of 500 milliseconds per division, and the bottom is 50 milliseconds per division. The right lower windows demonstrate the lack of identical superimposition caused by the instability.

Table 5
Disorders associated with unstable motor unit potentials

Type of Disease	Examples
Anterior horn cell diseases (with ongoing reinnervation)	ALS, spinal muscular atrophy, spinobulbar muscular atrophy
Radiculopathies	Recovering or ongoing reinnervation
Plexopathies	Recovering or ongoing reinnervation
Mononeuropathies	Recovering or ongoing reinnervation
Polyneuropathies (axonal)	Axonal neuropathies
Myopathies (uncommon)	Chronic, with reinnervation of fibers
Neuromuscular junction disorders	Myasthenia gravis, Lambert-Eaton myasthenic syndrome, congenital myasthenic syndromes, botulism, botulinum toxin administration

composed of a few or many action potentials, and the group morphology does not change as it fires repeatedly. There may be sudden shifts in firing rate or number of spikes within the group, and abrupt onsets or cessations of the CRD. The repetition rate of the group of spikes varies widely and may be as slow as 1 Hz or as fast as 150 Hz.[7,9] The individual spikes within a group are generated from ephaptic spread of action potentials to adjacent muscle fibers (**Fig. 14**). CRDs are nonspecific; they are commonly found in chronic neurogenic and myopathic disorders[55–57] (**Table 6**).

Long-Duration, High-Amplitude Motor Unit Potentials

Long-duration, high-amplitude MUPs result from the summation of more muscle fiber action potentials caused by increased fiber density from reinnervation. Their presence suggests longstanding reinnervation (more than several months) and are indicative of chronic or old neurogenic processes (**Table 7**). Long-duration, high-amplitude MUPs can also occur in chronic, or longstanding myopathies, likely because of chronic reinnervation of injured muscle fibers.

CASE 7. MYOKYMIC AND NEUROMYOTONIC DISCHARGES

A 39-year-old man was referred for evaluation of 1 year of muscle stiffness and gait difficulties. His NCS were normal. Needle EMG demonstrated myokymic discharges and neuromyotonic discharges in multiple leg and arm muscles.

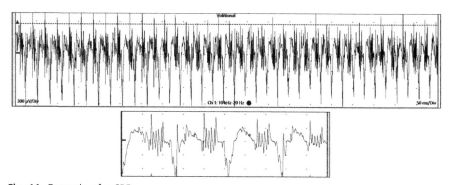

Fig. 14. Example of a CRD.

Table 6	
Disorders associated with complex repetitive discharges	
Type of Disease	**Examples**
Anterior horn cell diseases	ALS, spinal muscular atrophy, polio
Radiculopathies	Old or chronic
Plexopathies	Old or chronic
Mononeuropathies	Old or chronic
Polyneuropathies (axonal)	Old or chronic
Myopathies (chronic, with reinnervation)	Inclusion body myositis, muscular dystrophies

Myokymic Discharges

Myokymic discharges are uncommon spontaneous discharges that represent the spontaneous repeated firing of a motor unit in a burst firing pattern. Each burst is composed of one, or occasionally a few MUPs, and each burst recurs in a regular, semirhythmic, or sometimes irregular pattern. The firing frequencies within a burst and between bursts vary widely, although the firing rates within each burst are typically less than 150 Hz.[58,59] (**Fig. 15**) Myokymic discharges result from hyperexcitability of an anterior horn cell, brainstem nucleus, or axon, producing an ectopic generator at those levels.[58,60] They have been reported in various neurogenic disorders and are classically associated with focal nerve injury from radiation injury.[58,60,61] (**Table 8**)

Neuromyotonic Discharges

Neuromyotonic discharges are spontaneously firing discharges that are generated from recurrent, rapid firing of a motor unit at high rates of greater than 150 Hz.[7,58] The rate may remain relatively constant or increase or decrease rapidly. Neuromyotonic discharges may fire in long continuous runs or in intermittent bursts. When firing in bursts, the discharges are similar to myokymic discharges and may be differentiated by firing rates within a burst of greater than 150 Hz, whereas myokymic discharges fire at rates less than 150 Hz.[62] Neuromyotonic discharges occur as a result of anterior horn cell or axon hyperexcitability, and, when diffuse, are indicative of a peripheral nerve hyperexcitable disorder such as Isaac syndrome[63] (see **Table 8**).

Table 7	
Disorders associated with long-duration, high-amplitude motor unit potentials	
Type of Disease	**Examples**
Anterior horn cell diseases	ALS, spinal muscular atrophy, polio
Radiculopathies (old or chronic)	
Plexopathies (old or chronic)	
Mononeuropathies (old or chronic)	
Polyneuropathies (old or chronic)	Axonal neuropathies
Myopathies (chronic, with reinnervation)	Inclusion body myositis

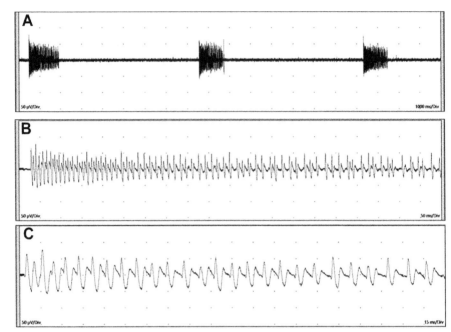

Fig. 15. Example of myokymic discharge at different display sweeps. (*A*) Sweep of 1 second/ division demonstrates the burst pattern of firing of 3 bursts. (*B*) Sweep of 50 milliseconds per division, and (*C*) sweep of 15 milliseconds per division show the same MUP firing repetitively within a single burst.

Table 8	
Disorders associated with myokymic and neuromyotonic discharges	
Type of Disease	**Examples**
Myokymic	
Radiation nerve injury	Plexopathy, mononeuropathy, cranial neuropathy
Chronic neurogenic disorders	Mononeuropathies (eg, carpal tunnel syndrome) Radiculopathies Polyradiculopathies Bell palsy Amyotrophic lateral sclerosis
Peripheral nerve hyperexcitable disorders	Isaac syndrome Morvan syndrome
Central nervous system disorders	Multiple sclerosis Brainstem neoplasms
Neuromyotonic	
Peripheral nerve hyperexcitable disorders	Isaac syndrome Morvan syndrome Episodic ataxia type 1
Hereditary neuropathies	HINT1 axonal neuropathy Spinal muscular atrophy

SUMMARY

The various EMG waveforms that are recorded during needle EMG, in isolation and in association with MUP changes, help to define the type of neuromuscular (or central) process that may be present and determine the temporal course and severity of the condition. Accurate recognition and interpretation of EMG waveforms is a critical component of an EDX medicine examination, which, when used in conjunction with NCS, helps to formulate a differential diagnosis to better determine the underlying etiology of the disease.

CLINICS CARE POINTS

- Identifying the firing pattern (regular, irregular, or semirhythmic) of each recurring waveform is necessary to identify the waveform
- Fibrillation potentials fire in a regular firing pattern, may have a spike or positive wave morphology, and are markers of denervated muscle fibers; they are nonspecific and can occur in various neuromuscular disorders.
- Fasciculation potentials and myotonic, myokymic, and neuromyotonic discharges are spontaneous waveforms with different firing patterns and rates of spike recurrence; their presence may be helpful in narrowing the differential diagnosis of the etiology of the disorder.
- Various changes in recruitment of MUPs and the configuration (phases, stability, duration, area, amplitude) of the MUPs occur over time following an acute neurogenic process; identification of these changes can help to determine the chronicity of the underlying process.

REFERENCES

1. Stalberg E, Nandedkar SD, Sanders DB, et al. Quantitative motor unit potential analysis. J Clin Neurophysiol 1996;13:401–22.
2. Bischoff C, Stalberg E, Falck B, et al. Reference values of motor unit action potentials obtained with multi-MUAP analysis. Muscle Nerve 1994;17:842–51.
3. Boe SG, Stashuk DW, Brown WF, et al. Decomposition-based quantitative electromyography: effect of force on motor unit potentials and motor unit number estimates. Muscle Nerve 2005;31:365–73.
4. Fuglsang-Frederiksen A. The utility of interference pattern analysis. Muscle Nerve 2000;23:18–36.
5. Barkhaus PE, Nandedkar SD. Quantitative EMG in inflammatory myopathies. Muscle Nerve 1990;13:247–53.
6. Boe SG, Antonowicz NM, Leung VW, et al. High inter-rater reliability in analyzing results of decomposition based quantitative electromyography in subjects with or without neuromuscular disorder. J Neurosci Methods 1992;192:138–45.
7. Daube JR, Rubin DI. Needle electromyography. Muscle Nerve 2009;39:244–70.
8. Rubin DI. Needle electromyography: basic concepts and patterns of abnormalities. Neurol Clin 2012;30:429–56.
9. Stålberg E, van Dijk H, Falck B, et al. Standards for quantification of EMG and neurography. Clin Neurophysiol 2019;130:1688–729.
10. Dumitru D, King JC, Stegeman DF. Normal needle electromyographic insertional activity morphology: a clinical and simulation study. Muscle Nerve 1998;21:910–20.

11. Wiechers DO, Stow R, Johnson EW. Electromyographic insertional activity mechanically provoked in the biceps brachii. Arch Phys Med Rehabil 1977;58: 573–8.
12. Wiechers DO. Electromyographic insertional activity in normal limb muscles. Arch Phys Med Rehabil 1979;60:359–63.
13. Wiechers DO. Mechanically provoked insertional activity before and after nerve section in rats. Arch Phys Med Rehabil 1977;58:402–5.
14. Wilbourn AJ. An unreported, distinctive type of increased insertional activity. Muscle Nerve 1982;5:S101–5.
15. Chow DW, Slipman CW, Ellen M, et al. "EMG disease" with bulbar muscle involvement: a case report. Arch Phys Med Rehabil 2002;83:568–9.
16. Young NP, Daube JR, Sorenson EJ, et al. Absent, unrecognized, and minimal myotonic discharges in myotonic dystrophy type 2. Muscle Nerve 2010;41: 758–62.
17. Mitchell CW, Bertorini TE. Diffusely increased insertional activity: "EMG disease" or asymptomatic myotonia congenita? A report of 2 cases. Arch Phys Med Rehabil 2007;88:1212–3.
18. Nam TS, Jung HJ, Choi SY, et al. Clinical characteristics and analysis of CLCN1 in patients with "EMG disease". J Clin Neurol 2012;8:212–7.
19. Johnson EW, Melvin JL. Value of electromyography in lumbar radiculopathy. Arch Phys Med Rehabil 1971;52:239–43.
20. Buchthal F, Rosenfalck P. Spontaneous electrical activity of human muscle. Electroencephalogr Clin Neurophysiol 1966;20:321–36.
21. Brown WF, Varkey GP. The origin of spontaneous electrical activity at the endplate zone. Ann Neurol 1981;10:557.
22. Dumitru D, King JC, Stegeman DF. Endplate spike morphology: a clinical and simulation study. Arch Phys Med Rehabil 1998;79:634–40.
23. Li CL, Shy GM, Wells J. Some properties of mammalian skeletal muscle fibres with particular reference to fibrillation potentials. J Physiol 1957;135:522–35.
24. Purves D, Sakman B. Membrane properties underlying spontaneous activity of denervated muscle fibres. J Physiol 1974;239:58–66.
25. Desmedt JE. Muscular dystrophy contrasted with denervation: different mechanisms underlying spontaneous fibrillations. Contemp Clin Neurophysiol 1978;(34):531–46.
26. Willmott AD, White C, Dukelow SP. Fibrillation potential onset in peripheral nerve injury. Muscle and Nerve 2012;48:332–40.
27. Dumitru D. Configuration of normal and abnormal non-volitional single muscle fiber discharges. Clin Neurophysiol 2000;111:1400–10.
28. Dumitru D, King JC. Hybrid fibrillation potentials and positive sharp waves. Muscle Nerve 2000;23:1234–42.
29. Rubin DI, Dimberg EL. Needle EMG of thenar muscles in less severe carpal tunnel syndrome. J Clin Neurophysiol 2018;35:481–4.
30. Sener U, Martinez-Thompson J, Laughlin RS, et al. Needle electromyography and histopathologic correlation in myopathies. Muscle Nerve 2019;59:315–20.
31. De Luca CJ, LeFever RS, McCue MP, et al. Behaviour of human motor units in different muscles during linearly varying contractions. J Physiol 1982;329: 113–28.
32. Petajan JH. AAEM minimonograph #3: motor unit recruitment. Muscle Nerve 1991;14:489–502.
33. Daube JR. Electrodiagnostic studies in amyotrophic lateral sclerosis and other motor neuron disorders. Muscle Nerve 2000;23:1488–502.

34. Campos C, Malanda A, Gila L, et al. Quantification of jiggle in real electromyographic signals. Muscle Nerve 2000;23:1022–34.
35. Stalberg E, Andreassen S, Falck B, et al. Quantitative analysis of individual motor unit potentials: a proposition for standardized terminology and criteria for measurement. J Clin Neurophysiol 1986;3:313–48.
36. Borenstein S, Desmedt JE. Range of variations in motor unit potentials during reinnervation after traumatic nerve lesions in humans. Ann Neurol 1980;8:460–7.
37. Nandedkar S, Sanders DB, Stalberg EV, et al. Simulation of concentric needle EMG motor unit action potentials. Muscle Nerve 1988;11:151–9.
38. Sonoo M. New attempts to quantify concentric needle electromyography. Muscle Nerve 2002;(Suppl 11):S98–102.
39. Sonoo M, Stålberg E. The ability of MUP parameters to discriminate between normal and neurogenic MUPs in concentric EMG: analysis of the MUP "thickness" and the proposal of "size index. Electroencephalogr Clin Neurophysiol 1993;89:291–303.
40. de Carvalho M, Dengler R, Eisen A, et al. Electrodiagnostic criteria for diagnosis of ALS. Clin Neurophysiol 2008;119:497–503.
41. Sun TY, Chen JJ, Lin TS. Analysis of motor unit firing patterns in patients with central or peripheral lesions using singular-value decomposition. Muscle Nerve 2000; 23:1057–68.
42. Krarup C, Boeckstyns M, Ibsen A, et al. Remodeling of motor units after nerve regeneration studied by quantitative electromyography. Clin Neurophsyiology 2016;127:1675–82.
43. Stalberg E. Electrophysiological studies of reinnervation in amyotrophic lateral sclerosis. In: Rowland LP, editor. Human motor neuorn diseases. New York: Raven Press; 1982. p. 47–57.
44. Brumlik J, Drechsler B, Vannin T. The myotonic discharge in various neurological syndromes; a neurophysiological analysis. Electromyography 1970;4:369–83.
45. Raja Rayan DL, Hanna MG. Skeletal muscle channelopathies: nondystrophic myotonias and periodic paralysis. Curr Opin Neurol 2010;23:466–76.
46. Burge JA, Hanna MG. Novel insights into the pathomechanisms of skeletal muscle channelopathies. Curr Neurol Neurosci Rep 2012;12:62–9.
47. Barkhaus PE, Nandedkar SD. 'Slow' myotonic discharges. Muscle and Nerve 2006;34:799–800.
48. Streib EW, Sun SF. Distribution of electrical myotonia in myotonic muscular dystrophy. Ann Neurol 1983;14:80–2.
49. Streib EW. AAEE minimonograph #27: differential diagnosis of myotonic syndromes. Muscle Nerve 1987;10:603–15.
50. Kugelberg E. Electromyography in muscular dystrophies. Differentiation between dystrophies and chronic lower motor neuron lesions. J Neurol Neurosurg Psychiatry 1949;12:129–36.
51. Buchthal F. Electrophysiological signs of myopathy as related with muscle biopsy. Acta Neurol (Napoli) 1977;32:1–29.
52. Liguori R, Fuglsang-Frederiksen A, Nix W, et al. Electromyography in myopathy. Neurophysiol Clin 1997;27:200–3.
53. Stålberg E, Karlsson L. Simulation of EMG in pathological situations. Clin Neurophysiol 2001;112:869–78.
54. Harvey AM, Masland RL. The electromyogram in myasthenia gravis. Bull Johns Hopkins Hops 1941;48:1–13.
55. Meyer BU, Benecke R, Frank B, et al. Complex repetitive discharges in the iliopsoas muscle. J Neurol 1988;235:411–4.

56. Emeryk B, Hausmanova-Petrusewicz I, Nowak T. Spontaneous volleys of bizarre high-frequency potentials in neuro-muscular diseases. Electromyogr Clin Neurophysiol 1974;14:303–12.
57. Fellows LK, Foster BJ, Foster BJ, et al. Clinical significance of complex repetitive discharges: a case-control study. Muscle Nerve 2003;28:504–7.
58. Gutmann L, Gutmann L. Myokymia and neuromyotonia. J Neurol 2004;251: 138–42.
59. Gutmann L. AAEM minimonograph #37: facial and limb myokymia. Muscle Nerve 1991;14:1043–9.
60. Albers JW, Allen AA, Bastron JA, et al. Limb myokymia. Muscle Nerve 1981;4: 494–504.
61. Oishi T, Ryan CS, Vazquez do Campo R, et al. Quantitative analysis of myokymic discharges in radiation versus non-radiation cases. Muscle Nerve 2021;63(6): 861–7.
62. Daube JR. Myokymia and neuromyotonia. Muscle Nerve 2001;24:1711–2.
63. Maddison P, Mills KR, Newsom-Davis J. Clinical electrophysiological characterization of the acquired neuromyotonia phenotype of autoimmune peripheral nerve hyperexcitability. Muscle Nerve 2006;33:801–8.

Electrodiagnosis of Common Mononeuropathies

Median, Ulnar, and Fibular (Peroneal) Neuropathies

Kamakshi Patel, MD[a], Holli A. Horak, MD[b],*

KEYWORDS

- Median nerve • Ulnar nerve • Fibular nerve • Peroneal nerve • Mononeuropathy
- Carpal tunnel syndrome • Ulnar neuropathy at the elbow

KEY POINTS

- Standard electrodiagnostic techniques are recommended for the initial assessment of common mononeuropathies.
- Electrodiagnostic studies, including routine nerve conduction studies and comparison studies with higher sensitivity, are useful to assess for carpal tunnel syndrome or median mononeuropathy at the wrist.
- Ulnar neuropathy at the elbow diagnosis may require short segment stimulation analysis across the elbow.
- Fibular nerve entrapment may affect the common fibular nerve, but instances of isolated deep fibular or superficial fibular neuropathy may occur.
- Neuromuscular ultrasound examination has become an important tool to evaluate compressive mononeuropathies; neuromuscular ultrasound examination adds sensitivity and can evaluate for anatomic abnormalities contributing to a mononeuropathy.

INTRODUCTION

Several peripheral nerves are prone to compression at entrapment sites, including the median nerve at the wrist, ulnar nerve neuropathy at the elbow (UNE), and fibular (peroneal) nerve at the fibular head. Compression may occur when a nerve is superficial, neighboring a bony structure, pulled or stretched from repetitive use of a limb, or entrapped by overlying structures (eg, transverse carpal ligament). Other factors,

The author has nothing to disclose.
[a] University of Texas Medical Branch (UTMB), 301 University Boulevard, JSA 9.128, Galveston, TX 77555, USA; [b] University of Arizona College of Medicine- Tucson, 1501 North Campbell Avenue, Room 6212a, Tucson, AZ 87524, USA
* Corresponding author.
E-mail address: hhorak@email.arizona.edu

Neurol Clin 39 (2021) 939–955
https://doi.org/10.1016/j.ncl.2021.06.004

such as associated weight loss in fibular (peroneal) neuropathies or diabetes, may predispose a nerve to compression. Electrodiagnosis (EDX) studies are useful tools in the evaluation of compressive mononeuropathies. EDX testing can confirm the presence of injury to a nerve, localize the site of injury along the nerve, determine the severity of the injury, and determine the degree of recovery, all of which are valuable in the diagnosis and management of mononeuropathies. This article reviews the EDX assessment and features of the most common compressive mononeuropathies.

MEDIAN NEUROPATHY AT THE WRIST (CARPAL TUNNEL SYNDROME)

Median neuropathy at the wrist is the most common compressive neuropathy encountered in neuromuscular clinics, with an incidence of 376 per 100,000 person-years.[1] The median nerve originates from the ventral rami of the C5 to T1 cervical roots. Sensory fibers course to the spinal cord through the lateral cord, upper and middle trunks, and C6 to C7 roots. Motor fibers are derived from the C6 to T1 roots, with the innervation to the thenar eminence muscles derived from the C8 to T1 roots, lower trunk, and medial cord (**Fig. 1**). The nerve supplies several forearm muscles before coursing through the carpal tunnel at the wrist, between the flexor retinaculum and the carpal bones.[1,2] The nerve divides and gives off the recurrent motor branch, which innervates the thenar muscles, and continues in the hand to innervate the first 2 lumbricals. Sensory fibers form the digital cutaneous nerves to the first 3, and the lateral one-half of the fourth digits.[1,2]

Compression of the median nerve within the carpal tunnel may cause carpal tunnel syndrome (CTS), with patients experiencing numbness, tingling, burning, and/or pain within the median dermatomal distribution. Predisposing factors for compression include rheumatoid arthritis, ganglion cysts, osteophytes, hereditary neuropathy with liability to pressure palsies, and other medical conditions such as diabetes, pregnancy, hypothyroidism, acromegaly, and amyloidosis.

Role of Electrodiagnostic Evaluation

CTS is a clinically defined syndrome, but EDX studies are important to confirm a process involving the median nerve at the wrist, assess the severity of nerve injury, exclude other mimicking disorders such as cervical radiculopathy or proximal median neuropathy, and evaluate for other superimposed processes, such as a more diffuse polyneuropathy.[1] Although EDX is sensitive for detecting injury to the median nerve at the wrist, approximately 5% to 25% of patients who meet the clinical criteria for CTS have normal routine EDX studies.[3–5] In patients with clinically suspected CTS in whom routine nerve conduction studies (NCS) are normal, more advanced studies, including comparison studies, increase the sensitivity for detecting mild CTS.[4–6] Although additional studies increase the sensitivity, the risk for false positives is also increased and may be between 5% and 46%.[1,5,7]

The hallmark EDX features in CTS is focal nerve slowing, indicating demyelinating, at the wrist, which is identified by prolonged distal latencies or slowed conduction velocities in the distal nerve segments of sensory (and often motor) nerves. A comprehensive CTS practice parameter from 2002 reviews the EDX protocol for evaluating CTS.[5] Using this protocol, a sensitivity of 85% and specificity of 95% can be achieved in diagnosing CTS.[5] Many EDX studies are available to assess CTS, and in most cases the routine sensory and motor NCS are sufficient to establish the diagnosis[4,8,9] (**Table 1**). However, in some circumstances, routine studies do not identify focal slowing and more advanced techniques or calculated indices can be used.[4,6] No single technique or index has been shown to be superior to others.[9]

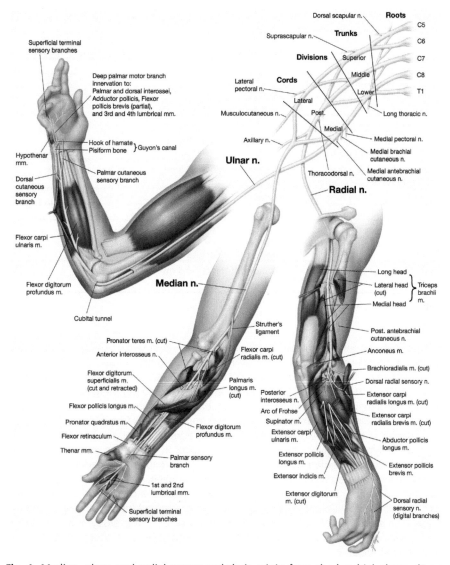

Fig. 1. Median, ulnar, and radial nerves and their origin from the brachial plexus. (*From* Dimberg EL. "Electrodiagnostic Evaluation of Ulnar Neuropathy and Other Upper Extremity Mononeuropathies." Neurol Clin 30 (2012), 479-503 as modified from the original (Neurology board review: an illustrated study guide. Rochester [MN]: Mayo Clinic Scientific Press and Boca Raton: Informa Healthcare USA; 2008); used with permission of Mayo Foundation for Medical Education and Research, all rights reserved.)

Routine Nerve Conduction Studies

Routine median motor NCS, recording from the thenar muscles, are performed to establish the presence of demyelination of the median nerve at wrist and assess disease severity.[1,5] Prolonged distal latencies with no or minimal conduction velocities slowing in the forearm localizes the lesion to the carpal tunnel, in the absence of similar

Table 1
Studies used to evaluate for CTS

	ABN Value[a]	Sensitivity	Specificity
Sensory + mixed			
Median antidromic (digit 2)	Latency >3.6 ms Amplitude >15 μV Conduction velocities of >56 m/s	65%	98%
Orthodromic palmar study	Latency difference >0.3 ms	71%	97%
Median-ulnar (ring finger) antidromic (Ringdiff)	Latency difference >0.4 ms	85%	97%
Median-radial (thumb) antidromic (Thumbdiff)	Latency difference >0.5 ms	65%	99%
Combined sensory index (CSI)	>1 ms	83%	
Motor			
Median motor over APB	Latency >4.5 ms Amplitude <4 mV Conduction velocities of >48 m/s	63% 44%–55%	
Median-ulnar lumbrical vs interosseous study	Latency difference >0.5 ms		

[a] Reference values are laboratory dependent.

changes in other nerves.[1,5] In more severe disease characterized by axonal loss, low compound muscle action potential (CMAP) amplitudes may occur.

The median motor NCS are often normal in mild CTS, are less sensitive than median sensory NCS, and sensory NCS are almost always affected before motor NCS. There are multiple sensory or mixed NCS options, each with benefits and technical challenges. The median antidromic NCS, recording from the index finger, is a routine study and is useful to establish the integrity of sensory fibers.[5] Although distal latency prolongation is typical, polyneuropathy can also result in prolonged sensory DLs and comparison to nonmedian nerves is important.[1,5] Because the median antidromic NCS tests a longer nerve segment than midpalmar studies, in mild CTS with only slight focal demyelination, the sensitivity of antidromic studies is decreased . The median orthodromic mixed NCS assesses a shorter nerve segment (usually 8 cm), which increases the sensitivity of detecting mild slowing. However, this study has more technical challenges, such as stimulus artifact, which makes it more difficult than antidromic studies.

Advanced Techniques

Lumbrical recording
In patients with a severe median neuropathy at the wrist with degeneration of most or all axons, no CMAP response may be recorded from the thenar muscles. In this situation, localization to the wrist cannot be made because an absent response could also be seen with a more proximal median neuropathy. Detecting conduction slowing across the wrist can sometimes be accomplished by recording from second lumbrical (median innervated), because the fibers to that muscle are relatively spared compared with fibers to the thenar muscles. This technique compares the median CMAP latency from the second lumbrical to the ulnar CMAP latency recording from the second palmar interossei. A latency difference of greater than 0.5 ms is abnormal.[10–12]

Segmental palmar studies

The median NCS can also be performed with segmental, across palmar stimulation (**Fig. 2**). This testing is most useful in the context of a low amplitude median sensory nerve action potential (SNAP), because it may help to distinguish CTS from a more diffuse polyneuropathy. Because segments of the median nerve outside the carpal tunnel should conduct relatively normally in CTS, if both intracarpal and distal segments are abnormal, there is more likely a diffuse process such as neuropathy.[1] Also, in the presence of conduction block in the carpal tunnel, stimulation of the distal segment will yield a larger SNAP. Neuropraxia (focal segmental demyelination) is present if the amplitude of the proximal median SNAP is 50% or more of the distal SNAP.[1]

Short segment stimulation across the wrist

Sensory short segment stimulation ("inching") across wrist can be performed to assess very focal slowing or conduction block. Technical challenges include risk of stimulating overlapping sites and stimulation artifact. A peak latency difference of 0.5 ms or more between 2 inching sites is considered abnormal.[13]

Comparison Studies

Studies that compare the median sensory latencies with other nerves in the same hand are more sensitive in the diagnosis of CTS than only an absolute median nerve latency.[1,4,5,14,15] Comparison studies allow one to assess the focality of a median nerve injury using the patient as their own control. Comparison studies include median and ulnar antidromic (fourth digit recording), median and radial antidromic (thumb recording), and median–ulnar orthodromic (palmar) mixed NCS (see **Table 1**).

Combined sensory index

Multiple comparison studies can be combined into a sensory index (combined sensory index). Originally described by Robinson and colleagues,[7] this index is the sum of latency differences of the first digit (thumb) difference + fourth digit (ring) difference + palmar difference studies.[1] A sum of greater than 0.9 ms is abnormal. It has a reported sensitivity of 83% and specificity of 95%. However, because multiple comparisons are used to evaluate for focal entrapment, it increases the risk of a type 1 error (false positive). In contrast, if more than 1 finding is abnormal, it decreases the risk of type 1 error.[7]

Needle Electromyography

Needle electromyography (EMG) is important to help define the severity and degree of denervation, as well as to exclude other conditions such as proximal median neuropathy, cervical radiculopathy, or brachial plexopathy. Needle EMG of the thenar muscles is rarely abnormal if motor NCS are normal.[16] With severe CTS, needle EMG may assist with prognostication by assessing the degree of denervation (fibrillation potentials) and reinnervation.[5]

Carpal Tunnel Syndrome Grading

Many grading systems for assessing the severity of CTS have been developed using either EDX criteria alone or a combination of clinical and EDX criteria.[17–20] Most EDX grading scales incorporate the degree of sensory and motor NCS abnormalities, including the presence of conduction slowing (suggesting neuropraxis) or amplitude reduction (suggesting axonotmesis/neurotmesis). The grading systems have been questioned owing to a lack of correlation between the patient's clinical and electrophysiologic severity.[21] Treatment decisions should be based on clinical judgment and the consistent use of 1 system, rather than arbitrary applications. There is a

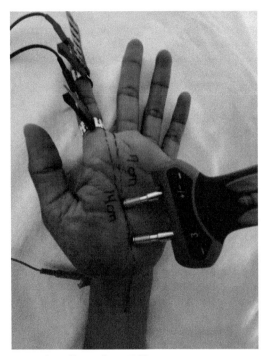

Fig. 2. Setup for segmental median palmar NCS.

positive correlation between CTS severity based on grading and improvement with surgical outcome.[6,17,22] A correlation between EDX severity and surgical outcome has also been shown.[8]

Electrodiagnostic Findings after Carpal Tunnel Syndrome Release

NCS are performed postoperatively in patients who have no clinical improvement after carpal tunnel release surgery or who develop symptoms again later in life. NCS may be important to evaluate for inadequate decompression or recurrence of entrapment. NCS are the only objective way to determine and quantify improvement after decompression. After surgery, improvement in electrophysiologic severity is seen in about 82% to 88% of patients at 6 to 9 months.[23] However, this finding may not correlate with symptom improvement. Sensory and motor latencies improve at 6 and 12 months respectively, but some slowing may persist in both latencies at 12 months in 80% of cases.[24] Because latencies improve but may not return to normal in most cases, recurrence of median nerve entrapment can only be diagnosed by comparing preoperative and postoperative NCS.

Neuromuscular Ultrasound Examination

Neuromuscular ultrasound (NMUS) examinations have become an important adjunct to EDX for evaluation of CTS. NMUS can confirm the diagnosis of CTS, detect mass lesions or structural abnormalities, and identify anatomic variants.[25–27] The cross-sectional area (CSA) of the nerve is measured at the wrist and a CSA ratio comparing wrist to forearm is calculated (**Fig. 3**). Many studies have shown a similar sensitivity and specificity of NMUS examination to EDX[26] and therefore NMUS examination is

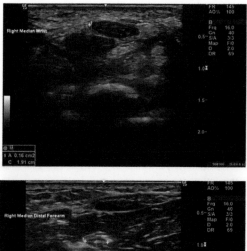

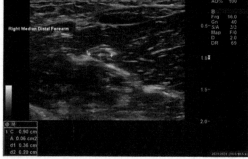

Fig. 3. Ultrasound examination of the median nerve at the wrist. (*Top*) Median nerve at the wrist. Enlarged median cross-sectional area (CSA) of 16 mm² at the wrist. (*Bottom*) Median nerve in forearm (CSA 6 mm²). (*Courtesy of* Katalin Scherer, MD.)

considered an adjunct to EDX studies.[26,27] In rare cases, NMUS examination may detect enlargement of the median nerve when EDX is normal.[27]

ULNAR NEUROPATHY

The ulnar nerve is the second most common mononeuropathy, and most commonly occurs owing to compression or subluxation at the elbow (UNE).[28] The ulnar nerve may be injured at the retrocondylar groove, humeroulnar arcade (ie, cubital tunnel), or, less commonly, at Guyon's canal at the wrist.[29–32] Although UNE can often be diagnosed by clinical examination, clinical localization is not always accurate.[28,33] Thus, EDX is an important tool to localize the site of nerve injury, assess severity, exclude other localizations (eg, C8 root or plexus), and help to guide management.[34,35]

The ulnar nerve derives from the C8 to T1 nerve roots, the lower trunk and medial cord.[28,33] There are no branches in the arm. The nerve passes in the retrocondylar groove and enters the cubital tunnel under the humeroulnar arcade approximately 2 to 3 cm distal to the medial epicondyle[30] (see **Fig. 1**; **Fig. 4**). In the forearm, the ulnar nerve innervates the medial portion of the flexor digitorum profundus (digits III and IV) and the flexor carpi ulnaris and gives off the dorsal ulnar cutaneous sensory branch, which supplies the dorsomedial hand.[30,32] At the wrist, it enters Guyon's canal, divides into a superficial branch (supplying the palmaris brevis muscle and the palmar sensation to the fifth and medial fourth digits), and a deep motor branch (innervating the ulnar hand muscles).[31,36]

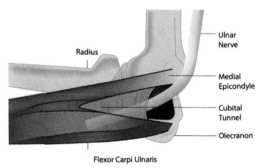

Fig. 4. Ulnar nerve at the elbow.

Patients with UNE present with subacute to chronic paresthesias of the fourth and fifth digits with some radiation into the hand. Although patients may perceive radiation into the forearm, objective sensory changes in the medial forearm sensory would indicate a more proximal localization (eg, medial cord/lower trunk or C8–T1 nerve root). The clinical findings of compression at Guyon's canal can seem similar to UNE, although sensation to the dorsum of the hand is spared.[31,36]

Role of Electrodiagnostic Evaluation

The goals of EDX testing in suspected UNE are to (1) confirm the presence of an ulnar neuropathy, (2) localize the site of injury along the nerve, (3) exclude other lesions/pathology such as polyneuropathy, C8 radiculopathy, or brachial plexopathy, (4) assess the pathophysiology (ie, demyelinating or axonal loss), (5) define the temporal course, and (6) define severity.[28,29] EDX studies have a high specificity but relatively low sensitivity for identifying UNE.[29,37,38]

NCS are the most useful techniques to confirm and localize an ulnar neuropathy[28,29,33] (**Table 2**). Routine ulnar motor and sensory NCS may be sufficient to identify the general region of nerve involvement, although advanced techniques (such as short segment studies) are often needed in mild cases or to more precisely localize the site of injury.[39] Although sensory NCS are usually affected earlier than motor NCS, motor NCS are more helpful to more precisely localize the injury around the elbow since they can better identify focal conduction block or a small latency shift.[29,32,36]

Routine Nerve Conduction Studies

Routine ulnar CMAPs are performed with recording from the abductor digiti minimi with stimulation at the wrist, below the elbow, and above the elbow sites.[29] The criteria for confirmation of UNE include absolute conduction velocities in the below the elbow–above the elbow segment less than 50 m/s or greater than 10 m/s slowing in the below the elbow–above the elbow segment compared with the wrist–below the elbow segment. A conduction block is suspected if the CMAP amplitude and area decreases by greater than 20% between below the elbow and above the elbow sites.[29,40] A recent study has highlighted statistical errors that may occur when strict diagnostic criteria are used; therefore, a graduated system based on pretest probability is recommended.[34,41,42]

The ulnar sensory antidromic NCS (recording fifth digit) assesses the ulnar sensory axons that course across the elbow. In demyelinating UNE, conduction velocity slowing in the sensory fibers may be seen; in more severe injury with axon loss, the SNAP amplitude is decreased. Sensory NCS findings are less useful at localizing the site of

Table 2
Electrodiagnostic findings in ulnar neuropathies and other mimickers

| | Ulnar Nerve | | | | |
	Deep Motor Branch (Hand)	Guyon's Canal	Elbow	Medial Cord/ Lower Trunk	C8 Root
NCS					
Ulnar motor (abductor digiti minimi)	N	ABN	ABN	ABN	ABN
Ulnar motor (first dorsal interosseous)	ABN	ABN	ABN	ABN	ABN
Ulnar sensory (fifth digit)	N	ABN	ABN	ABN	N
Dorsal ulnar cutaneous	N	N	ABN	ABN	N
Needle EMG					
First dorsal interosseous	ABN	ABN	ABN	ABN	ABN
Abductor digiti minimi	N	ABN	ABN	ABN	ABN
Flexor carpi ulnaris	N	N	May be ABN	ABN	ABN
Abductor policis brevis	N	N	N	ABN	ABN

Abbreviations: ABN, abnormal; N, normal.

injury along the nerve because the conduction block is more difficult to identify in sensory nerves. The ulnar SNAP may also be abnormal in lower trunk/medial cord plexopathies but is normal in C8/T1 radiculopathies. If Guyon's canal compression is suspected, the dorsal ulnar cutaneous sensory study should be performed.[29,36] In the setting of absent or decreased amplitude ulnar sensory antidromic studies, a normal dorsal ulnar cutaneous localizes the lesion at or distal to the wrist.

Advanced Nerve Conduction Studies

First dorsal interosseous recording
If no abnormality is identified on routine ulnar motor NCS recording from the abductor digiti minimi but the clinical suspicion is strong, recording from the first dorsal interosseous may increase sensitivity for detecting UNE.[28,41] In addition, abductor digiti minimi CMAPs may be normal in lesions affecting the deep palmar branch, but the first dorsal interosseous CMAPs will be affected. For suspected ulnar neuropathies at the wrist, ulnar CMAP to the first dorsal interosseous and dorsal ulnar cutaneous sensory are important to aid in localization.[29]

Short segment motor stimulation
A short segment study (inching) is a useful technique to localize more precisely the site of nerve compression by identifying a very focal area of demyelination, as identified by a focal latency shift or conduction block.[29] Several recent papers have evaluated the sensitivity and specificity of short segment studies.[40,42,43] Multiple studies have validated this technique, but have not agreed on the most common compression site; however, the most common site of maximal prolongation in latency or decrease in amplitude seems to be either just proximal or distal to the medial epicondyle[40,42,43] **(Fig. 5)**.

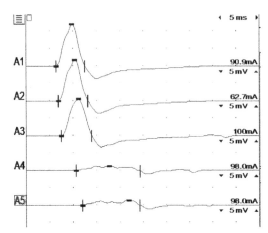

Fig. 5. Ulnar motor inching technique, showing a conduction block 1 cm proximal to medial epicondyle (between stimulation sites A3 and A4). (*Courtesy of* Devon Rubin, MD.)

Short segment sensory stimulation

In up to 20% of patients with clinical features consistent with mild UNE, routine NCS and even motor short segment studies may be insensitive to identify an abnormality.[40,42] Vazquez do Campo and colleagues[39] published a pilot study evaluating sensory 2-cm short segment studies across the elbow recording from the fifth digit, which improved the sensitivity of diagnosing UNE. Values of more than a 0.7-ms latency shift or a more than 15% decrease in amplitude were proposed.[39]

Needle Electromyography

Needle EMG is less helpful than NCS at precisely localizing the site of involvement along the ulnar nerve, but is useful to assess the severity and exclude other localizations (eg, C8 radiculopathy or brachial plexopathy).[29] Needle EMG is often normal if the underlying pathology is mild demyelination or only sensory fibers are involved. Needle EMG may demonstrate only decreased recruitment if there is focal conduction block without axonal loss, or fibrillation potentials and/or long duration motor unit potentials in axonal loss.[37,44] Proximal ulnar-innervated muscles (flexor carpi ulnaris or flexor digitorum profundus) may be normal on needle EMG owing to fascicular involvement or branching to those muscles proximal to the elbow.[28,29,44]

Neuromuscular Ultrasound Examination in Ulnar Nerve Neuropathy at the Elbow

NMUS examination can improve the sensitivity of diagnosing UNE.[25,38,42,45–47] An ulnar nerve circumference of more than 11 mm^2 or a ratio of ulnar nerve at the elbow to the wrist of more than 1.4 are considered abnormal[38,47] (**Fig. 6**). Ultrasound examination alone, without EDX, has been shown to have high sensitivity and specificity.[40,42] However, ultrasound examination does not provide information on severity or physiologic nerve function. Therefore, EDX and NMUS examination are complementary.[43,46]

FIBULAR (PERONEAL) NEUROPATHY

Compression of the common fibular nerve at the fibular head is the most common compression neuropathy of the lower extremity.[48–50] Causes include frequent leg crossing, prolonged kneeling, or significant weight loss (slimmer's palsy). Clinically,

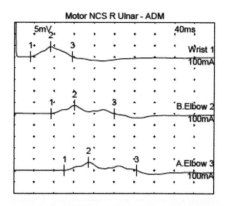

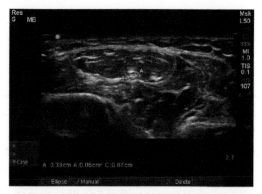

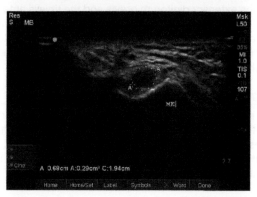

Fig. 6. Ulnar neuropathy at the elbow. (*Top*) Ulnar NCS with low amplitudes and temporal dispersion owing to axonal loss. (*Middle*) Ultrasound examination of the ulnar nerve under the flexor carpi ulnaris with normal CSA 5 mm². (*Bottom*) Enlarged ulnar nerve CSA of 29 mm² adjacent to the medial epicondyle. (*Courtesy of* Katalin Scherer, MD.)

patients present with weakness of foot dorsiflexion and eversion and numbness over the lateral leg and dorsum of foot.[50,51]

The fibular nerve contains axons originating in the L4 to L5 roots, which course through the lumbosacral plexus and sciatic nerve to form the common peroneal nerve

Table 3
Electrodiagnostic findings in fibular neuropathies and mimickers

	Fibular Neuropathy						
	Deep Fibular (Ankle)	Deep Fibular (Leg)	Superficial Fibular (Ankle)	Superficial Fibular (Leg)	Common Fibular	Sciatic Nerve	L5 Root
NCS							
Fibular motor (extensor digitorum brevis)	ABN	ABN	N	N	ABN	ABN	ABN
Fibular motor (AT)	N	ABN	N	N	ABN	ABN	ABN
Superficial fibular sensory	N	N	ABN	ABN	ABN	ABN	N
Needle electromyography							
Anterior tibialis	N	ABN	N	N	ABN	ABN	ABN
Peroneus longus/brevis	N	N	N	ABN	ABN	ABN	ABN
Biceps femoris, short head	N	N	N	N	N	ABN	ABN
Gluteus medius	N	N	N	N	N	N	ABN

Abbreviations: ABN, abnormal; AT, anterior tibialis; N, normal.

in the distal thigh. In the thigh, the fibular nerve gives off a branch to the short head of the biceps femoris and then courses posterior and distal to the fibular head, which is the most common site of compression.[50–52] The nerve divides into 2 branches, namely, the deep and superficial branches.[49,51] The deep branch innervates foot extensors, including the extensor digitorum brevis and the tibialis anterior, extensor digitorum longus, and peroneus tertius.[49] The superficial branch innervates the peroneus longus and brevis and divides into the medial and lateral dorsal cutaneous branches, supplying sensation to the entire dorsum of the foot, except for the first and second digit interspace, which is supplied by the deep fibular nerve.[49,52]

Role of Electrodiagnostic Testing

Electrodiagnostic evaluation of fibular neuropathy helps to confirm the diagnosis, localize the site of involvement along the nerve, determine which fibular branches are involved, assess severity, and exclude other localizations (eg, L5 radiculopathy or sciatic neuropathy)[1,48,53] (**Table 3**). A combination of NCS and needle EMG help to define those features.

Routine Nerve Conduction Studies

As discussed in the 2005 American Association of Neuromuscular Electrodiagnostic Medicine practice parameter, the fibular nerve EDX studies have not been standardized.[53–55] Injury to the common fibular nerve may cause focal demyelination, which is manifest on NCS as conduction velocities slowing or conduction block at the fibular head, or axonal loss, which is manifest by low amplitudes. If only the deep fibular branch is involved, motor NCS to the extensor digitorum brevis and/or tibialis anterior may be involved but superficial fibular sensory NCS will be spared. In contrast, superficial fibular neuropathies may have normal motor NCS but abnormal superficial fibular SNAP.[51,53,56]

The criteria for abnormality on the fibular motor NCS include greater than 20% drop in amplitude at the fibular head compared with the ankle.[44,50] Other studies use a combination of findings, including a 50% decrease in amplitude at the knee compared with distal amplitude or conduction velocity slowing of more than 10 m/s in the across fibular head segment (knee–fibular head) compared with below the fibular head segment (fibular head–ankle)[53,54,57](Fig. 7). If the CMAP amplitude at ankle is low (<2 mV), localization may be difficult because focal slowing or conduction block (CB) may not be identified.[53,54] Recording from the tibialis anterior, which may be relatively spared compared with the extensor digitorum brevis, may assist in identifying focal slowing or CB at the fibular head.[51,53]

The superficial fibular sensory NCS will be the only sensory NCS that is abnormal in fibular neuropathies characterized by axonal loss and involving the common or superficial fibular nerves, but will be spared in conditions involving only the deep branch.[54,56] Furthermore, in common fibular neuropathies characterized by CB, the superficial fibular SNAP may be normal because stimulation is usually performed at a site distal to the block.[53,56]

Needle Electromyography

Needle EMG helps to define the temporal course of the injury, severity, degree of axonal loss, and degree of reinnervation.[48,51] Needle examination of muscles supplied by the deep and superficial branches is important to localize the lesion. Furthermore, when all fibular leg muscles are abnormal and focal slowing or block is not identified at the fibular head, examination of the short head of the biceps femoris is important to identify the most proximal site of the injury. Because all fibular muscles are supplied by the L5 root, other nonfibular L5 muscles should be examined to exclude an L5 radiculopathy.

Advanced Studies

Short segment stimulation
Short segment stimulation (inching) with stimulation in 2-cm segments across the fibular head may be more sensitive than routine NCS in identifying focal slowing.[55] Inching can be performed recording from the extensor digitorum brevis or the tibialis anterior.

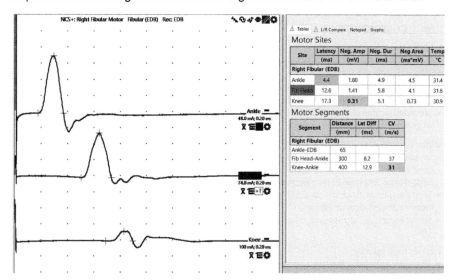

Motor Sites

Site	Latency (ms)	Neg. Amp (mV)	Neg. Dur (ms)	Neg Area (ms*mV)	Temp °C
Right Fibular (EDB)					
Ankle	4.4	1.80	4.9	4.5	31.4
Fib Head	12.6	1.41	5.8	4.1	31.6
Knee	17.3	0.31	5.1	0.73	30.9

Motor Segments

Segment	Distance (mm)	Lat Diff (ms)	CV (m/s)
Right Fibular (EDB)			
Ankle-EDB	65		
Fib Head-Ankle	300	8.2	37
Knee-Ankle	400	12.9	31

Fig. 7. Fibular motor NCS demonstrating a conduction block at the fibular head.

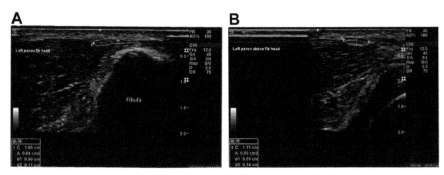

Fig. 8. Ultrasound examination of a normal fibular nerve at (*A*) fibular head (nerve CSA 4 mm²) and (*B*) the knee (nerve CSA 6 mm²). (*Courtesy of* Katalin Scherer, MD.)

Neuromuscular Ultrasound Examination

Ultrasound examination, assessing the CSA of the nerve at the fibular head, can complement EDX testing, and enlargement of the fibular CSA supports a fibular mononeuropathy[50,57] (**Fig. 8**). Furthermore, NMUS examination can occasionally identify structural processes as the cause of the fibular neuropathy.[57,58] Ganglion cysts have been reported to occur in up to 18% of confirmed fibular neuropathy.[58]

SUMMARY

The median, ulnar, and fibular nerves are the most commonly injured peripheral nerves. Electrodiagnostic testing plays an important role in assessing these mononeuropathies. Although routinely performed NCS and needle EMG studies may be sufficient to provide the necessary localization and information about the nerve function, in some case, more advanced techniques are necessary. The addition of NMUS examination promises to assist with localization and demonstration of any potential underlying structural abnormality.

CLINICS CARE POINTS

Median Neuropathy:
- Comparison studies can be more sensitive than routine nerve conduction studies in diagnosing carpal tunnel syndrome.
- Neuromuscular ultrasound can be used to confirm, diagnose or evaluate for any structural etiologies for median neuropathy at the wrist.

Ulnar neuropathy:
- In patients with a strong clinical suspicion of ulnar neuropathy at the elbow and normal routine ulnar motor study with recording from Abductor digiti minimi, recording from First dorsal interrossei may increase sensitivity.
- Short segment (inching studies) is a useful technique to precisely localize the site of ulnar nerve compression at elbow.
- Neuromuscular ultrasound is an useful adjunct test to improve sensitivity for diagnosing UNE.

Fibular neuropathy:
- The fibular head is the most common site of compression for common fibular neuropathies, but sometimes isolated superficial or deep branches of the peroneal nerve may be involved.

• Neuromuscular ultrasound can complement EDX testing and may help identify structural processes like ganglion cysts as cause of fibular neuropathies.

ACKNOWLEDGMENTS

The authors thank Katalin Scherer, MD for obtaining and lending ultrasound and waveform images used in this article, Devon Rubin, MD for lending images, his advice and editing and Monique Garcia for help with images.

REFERENCES

1. Werner RA, Andary M. Electrodiagnostic evaluation of carpal tunnel syndrome. Muscle Nerve 2011;44(4):597–607.
2. Hobson-Webb LD, Juel VC. Common entrapment neuropathies. Continuum (Minneap Minn) 2017;23(2, Selected Topics in Outpatient Neurology):487–511.
3. Witt JC, Hentz JG, Stevens JC. Carpal tunnel syndrome with normal nerve conduction studies. Muscle Nerve 2004;29(4):515–22.
4. Zeidman LA, Singh SK, Pandey DK. Higher diagnostic yield with the combined sensory index in mild carpal tunnel syndrome. J Clin Neuromuscul Dis 2014; 15(4):143–6.
5. Jablecki CK, Andary MT, Floeter MK, et al. Practice parameter: electrodiagnostic studies in carpal tunnel syndrome. Report of the American Association of Electrodiagnostic Medicine, American Academy of Neurology, and the American Academy of Physical Medicine and Rehabilitation. Neurology 2002;58(11):1589–92.
6. Zeidman LA, Pandey DK. A carpal tunnel grading system including combined sensory index-diagnosed mild cases: relation to presenting features and outcomes. Muscle Nerve 2018;57(1):45–8.
7. Robinson LR, Micklesen PJ, Wang L. Optimizing the number of tests for carpal tunnel syndrome. Muscle Nerve 2000;23(12):1880–2.
8. Bland JD. Do nerve conduction studies predict the outcome of carpal tunnel decompression? Muscle Nerve 2001;24(7):935–40.
9. Keith MW, Masear V, Chung K, et al. Diagnosis of carpal tunnel syndrome. J Am Acad Orthop Surg 2009;17(6):389–96.
10. Preston DC, Logigian EL. Lumbrical and interossei recording in carpal tunnel syndrome. Muscle Nerve 1992;15(11):1253–7.
11. Muellbacher W, Mamoli B, Zifko U, et al. Lumbrical and interossei recording in carpal tunnel syndrome. Muscle Nerve 1994;17(3):359–60.
12. Trojaborg W, Grewal RP, Weimer LH, et al. Value of latency measurements to the small palm muscles compared to other conduction parameters in the carpal tunnel syndrome. Muscle Nerve 1996;19(2):243–5.
13. Nathan PA, Keniston RC, Meadows KD, et al. Predictive value of nerve conduction measurements at the carpal tunnel. Muscle Nerve 1993;16(12):1377–82.
14. Alemdar M. Ring finger sensorial conduction studies in grading carpal tunnel syndrome. J Back Musculoskelet Rehabil 2016;29(2):309–15.
15. Alemdar M. Ring finger sensorial conduction studies in grading carpal tunnel syndrome: part II. J Back Musculoskelet Rehabil 2018;31(4):759–66.
16. Rubin DI, Dimberg EL. Needle EMG of thenar muscles in less severe carpal tunnel syndrome. J Clin Neurophysiol 2018;35(6):481–4.
17. Hirani S. A study to further develop and refine carpal tunnel syndrome (CTS) nerve conduction grading tool. BMC Musculoskelet Disord 2019;20(1):581.

18. Noszczyk BH, Nowak M, Krzesniak N. Use of the accordion severity grading system for negative outcomes of carpal tunnel syndrome. J Plast Reconstr Aesthet Surg 2013;66(8):1123–30.

19. Padua L, LoMonaco M, Gregori B, et al. Neurophysiological classification and sensitivity in 500 carpal tunnel syndrome hands. Acta Neurol Scand 1997; 96(4):211–7.

20. Bland JD. A neurophysiological grading scale for carpal tunnel syndrome. Muscle Nerve 2000;23(8):1280–3.

21. Chan L, Turner JA, Comstock BA, et al. The relationship between electrodiagnostic findings and patient symptoms and function in carpal tunnel syndrome. Arch Phys Med Rehabil 2007;88(1):19–24.

22. Park KM, Shin KJ, Park J, et al. The usefulness of terminal latency index of median nerve and f-wave difference between median and ulnar nerves in assessing the severity of carpal tunnel syndrome. J Clin Neurophysiol 2014;31(2):162–8.

23. Tahririan MA, Moghtaderi A, Aran F. Changes in electrophysiological parameters after open carpal tunnel release. Adv Biomed Res 2012;1:46.

24. Prick JJ, Blaauw G, Vredeveld JW, et al. Results of carpal tunnel release. Eur J Neurol 2003;10(6):733–6.

25. Gonzalez NL, Hobson-Webb LD. Neuromuscular ultrasound in clinical practice: a review. Clin Neurophysiol Pract 2019;4:148–63.

26. Cartwright MS, Hobson-Webb LD, Boon AJ, et al. Evidence-based guideline: neuromuscular ultrasound for the diagnosis of carpal tunnel syndrome. Muscle Nerve 2012;46(2):287–93.

27. Aseem F, Williams JW, Walker FO, et al. Neuromuscular ultrasound in patients with carpal tunnel syndrome and normal nerve conduction studies. Muscle Nerve 2017;55(6):913–5.

28. Dimberg EL. Electrodiagnostic evaluation of ulnar neuropathy and other upper extremity mononeuropathies. Neurol Clin 2012;30(2):479–503.

29. Practice parameter for electrodiagnostic studies in ulnar neuropathy at the elbow: summary statement. American Association of Electrodiagnostic Medicine, American Academy of Neurology, American Academy of Physical Medicine and Rehabilitation. Muscle Nerve 1999;22(3):408–11.

30. Palmer BA, Hughes TB. Cubital tunnel syndrome. J Hand Surg Am 2010;35(1): 153–63.

31. Earp BE, Floyd WE, Louie D, et al. Ulnar nerve entrapment at the wrist. J Am Acad Orthop Surg 2014;22(11):699–706.

32. Shea JD, McClain EJ. Ulnar-nerve compression syndromes at and below the wrist. J Bone Joint Surg Am 1969;51(6):1095–103.

33. Strakowski J. Ultrasound evaluation of peripheral nerves and focal neuropathies. 2nd edition. New York: Springer; 2021.

34. Omejec G, Podnar S. Precise localization of ulnar neuropathy at the elbow. Clin Neurophysiol 2015;126(12):2390–6.

35. Osei DA, Groves AP, Bommarito K, et al. Cubital tunnel syndrome: incidence and demographics in a national administrative database. Neurosurgery 2017;80(3): 417–20.

36. Coraci D, Loreti C, Piccinini G, et al. Ulnar neuropathy at wrist: entrapment at a very "congested" site. Neurol Sci 2018;39(8):1325–31.

37. Walker FO, Cartwright MS, Alter KE, et al. Indications for neuromuscular ultrasound: expert opinion and review of the literature. Clin Neurophysiol 2018; 129(12):2658–79.

38. Cartwright MS, Demar S, Griffin LP, et al. Validity and reliability of nerve and muscle ultrasound. Muscle Nerve 2013;47(4):515–21.
39. Vazquez do Campo R, Dimberg E, Rubin D. Short segment sensory nerve stimulation in suspected ulnar neuropathy at the elbow: a pilot study. Muscle Nerve 2019;59(1):125–9.
40. Pelosi L, Tse DMY, Mulroy E, et al. Ulnar neuropathy with abnormal non-localizing electrophysiology: clinical, electrophysiological and ultrasound findings. Clin Neurophysiol 2018;129(10):2155–61.
41. Logigian EL, Villanueva R, Twydell PT, et al. Electrodiagnosis of ulnar neuropathy at the elbow (Une): a Bayesian approach. Muscle Nerve 2014;49(3):337–44.
42. Omejec G, Podnar S. Normative values for short-segment nerve conduction studies and ultrasonography of the ulnar nerve at the elbow. Muscle Nerve 2015;51(3):370–7.
43. Simon NG, Ralph JW, Poncelet AN, et al. A comparison of ultrasonographic and electrophysiologic 'inching' in ulnar neuropathy at the elbow. Clin Neurophysiol 2015;126(2):391–8.
44. Stalberg E, van Dijk H, Falck B, et al. Standards for quantification of EMG and neurography. Clin Neurophysiol 2019;130(9):1688–729.
45. Baute Penry V, Cartwright MS. Neuromuscular ultrasound for peripheral neuropathies. Semin Neurol 2019;39(5):542–8.
46. Alrajeh M, Preston DC. Neuromuscular ultrasound in electrically non-localizable ulnar neuropathy. Muscle Nerve 2018;58(5):655–9.
47. Cartwright MS, Passmore LV, Yoon JS, et al. Cross-sectional area reference values for nerve ultrasonography. Muscle Nerve 2008;37(5):566–71.
48. Fridman V, David WS. Electrodiagnostic evaluation of lower extremity mononeuropathies. Neurol Clin 2012;30(2):505–28.
49. Poage C, Roth C, Scott B. Peroneal nerve palsy: evaluation and management. J Am Acad Orthop Surg 2016;24(1):1–10.
50. Tsukamoto H, Granata G, Coraci D, et al. Ultrasound and neurophysiological correlation in common fibular nerve conduction block at fibular head. Clin Neurophysiol 2014;125(7):1491–5.
51. Stewart JD. Foot drop: where, why and what to do? Pract Neurol 2008;8(3):158–69.
52. Katirji B, Wilbourn AJ. High sciatic lesion mimicking peroneal neuropathy at the fibular head. J Neurol Sci 1994;121(2):172–5.
53. Marciniak C, Armon C, Wilson J, et al. Practice parameter: utility of electrodiagnostic techniques in evaluating patients with suspected peroneal neuropathy: an evidence-based review. Muscle Nerve 2005;31(4):520–7.
54. Karakis I, Khoshnoodi M, Liew W, et al. Electrophysiologic features of fibular neuropathy in childhood and adolescence. Muscle Nerve 2017;55(5):693–7.
55. Kanakamedala RV, Hong CZ. Peroneal nerve entrapment at the knee localized by short segment stimulation. Am J Phys Med Rehabil 1989;68(3):116–22.
56. Murad H, Neal P, Katirji B. Total innervation of the extensor digitorum brevis by the accessory deep peroneal nerve. Eur J Neurol 1999;6(3):371–3.
57. Visser LH, Hens V, Soethout M, et al. Diagnostic value of high-resolution sonography in common fibular neuropathy at the fibular head. Muscle Nerve 2013;48(2):171–8.
58. Cartwright MS, Walker FO. Neuromuscular ultrasound in common entrapment neuropathies. Muscle Nerve 2013;48(5):696–704.

Electrodiagnostic Assessment of Uncommon Mononeuropathies

Ghazala Hayat, MD[a],*, Jeffrey S. Calvin, MD[b]

KEYWORDS

- Axillary neuropathy • Musculocutaneous neuropathy • Suprascapular neuropathy
- Sciatic neuropathy • Obturator neuropathy • Proximal neuropathies of limbs
- Uncommon neuropathies

KEY POINTS

- Uncommon upper and lower extremities mononeuropathies may be challenging to diagnose because they may mimic disorders involving cervical or lumbosacral roots, plexopathies, or non-neuromuscular disorders.
- Electrodiagnostic studies play an important role in the diagnosis, localization, and prognosis of uncommon mononeuropathies.
- Knowledge of anatomy of nerves in the upper and lower extremities that are not routinely examined and performance of appropriate electrodiagnostic testing.
- In these technically difficult electrodiagnostic studies monitoring for technical problems is critical for accurate performance and interpretation of the studies.

INTRODUCTION

Carpal tunnel syndrome (CTS), ulnar neuropathy at the elbow, and peroneal neuropathy are the most common mononeuropathies; however other individual nerves in the upper extremities (UE) and lower extremities (LE) may also be injured by various processes. These uncommon mononeuropathies may be less readily diagnosed owing to unfamiliarity with the presentations and vague symptoms. Electrodiagnostic (EDX) studies are essential in the evaluation of uncommon mononeuropathies and can assist in localization and prognostication. However, they can also be challenging, because stimulation at the proximal sites is difficult and well-validated reference values are not available. This article reviews the EDX assessment of several uncommon UE and LE mononeuropathies.

The authors have no conflicts of interest to disclose.
[a] Saint Louis University School of Medicine, Saint Louis, MO, USA; [b] Department of Neurology, Saint Louis University School of Medicine, Saint Louis, MO, USA
* Corresponding author.
E-mail address: ghazala.hayat@health.slu.edu

PROXIMAL MEDIAN NEUROPATHY

Disorders involving the median nerve proximal to the wrist are much less common than median neuropathy at the wrist or CTS.[1] In a series from Cleveland Clinic, only 0.2% of patients referred for EDX had findings of a proximal median neuropathy.[2] The median nerve comprises of branches from the C5 to T1 roots derived from medial and lateral cords of the brachial plexus.[3] The nerve enters the arm in the axilla at the inferior margin of the teres major muscle, passes lateral to the brachial artery and between the biceps brachii and brachialis muscles (**Fig. 1**). It runs medial to the brachial artery in the distal arm into the cubital fossa, passing between the heads of the pronator teres (PT), and travels between the flexor digitorum superficialis (FDS) and flexor digitorum profundus (FDP) muscles. In the cubital fossa, it gives off branches to the flexor carpi radialis (FCR), palmaris longus (PL), and FDS muscles. The anterior interosseous branches from the median nerve in the upper forearm, innervating the flexor pollicis longus (FPL), lateral one-half of the FDP, and the pronator quadratus (PQ). In the forearm, the median nerve also gives off sensory branches, including the palmar cutaneous branch in the distal forearm, supplying sensation to the thenar eminence. It then enters the hand in the carpal tunnel, and supplies the muscles of the thenar eminence, as well as giving off digital branches to the thumb, index, middle, and lateral ring fingers.

Etiologies and Sites of Compression

Proximal median neuropathy can occur from diverse etiologies, including trauma, external compression from casting, venipuncture, tumors or hematoma, or as part of a more diffuse process such as Parsonage–Turner syndrome or multifocal motor neuropathy with conduction block.[1,4] Nerve entrapment can occur (1) in the upper

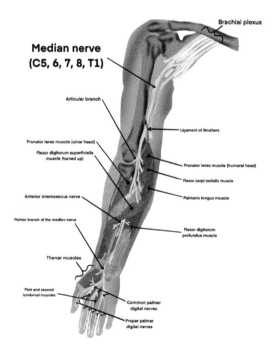

Fig. 1. Median nerve anatomy.

arm from a bony spur originating from the humeral shaft just proximal to the medial epicondyle, and a fibrous structure (ligament of Struthers) connecting the spur to the medial epicondyle[4–6]; (2) by a fibrous band (lacertus fibrosus) that runs between the forearm flexor muscles and the biceps tendon; (3) within the PT muscle, particularly with anatomic variants of additional fibrous bands within the muscle; or (4) beneath the sublimus bridge of the FDS muscle.

Clinical Features

The clinical features of proximal median neuropathies depend on the etiology and the specific site of the lesion.[2,7] In proximal lesions, sensory disturbance usually involves the entire median distribution, including the hand, and sensory loss of the proximal thenar eminence indicates a more proximal lesion than the wrist. The distribution of weakness also depends on the site of the lesion and may involve median innervated forearm and/or hand muscles.

Entrapment at the ligament of Struthers produces a syndrome characterized by pain and paresthesia in the volar surface of the forearm and the median innervated digits that is exacerbated by elbow extension or forearm supination. These positioning maneuvers may also attenuate the radial pulse because the brachial artery runs under the ligament of Struthers in the neurovascular bundle with the median nerve. Subtle sensory loss may occur over the thenar eminence and weakness may be seen in the median innervated muscles in the forearm. Features in pronator syndrome are nonspecific and often includes pain in the forearm that radiates proximally. A positive Tinel sign may be present over the PT muscle. Symptoms may be exacerbated by pronation–supination of the forearm. Mild weakness of the median-innervated muscles is not uncommon, but severe weakness is rare.

The anterior interosseous nerve (AION) syndrome presents with unique clinical features of weakness of thumb flexion, finger flexion for digits 2 and 3, and protonation, resulting in a "teardrop" shape when attempting to make an "OK" sign[8,9] (**Fig. 2**A, B). Although there may be deep forearm pain or subjective sensory symptoms, cutaneous sensation remains intact.

Electrophysiologic Features

EDX studies are useful to localize the site of lesion along the median nerve and exclude other localizations[2] (**Table 1**). In processes characterized by axon degeneration, the median motor nerve conduction studies recording from the abductor pollicis brevis

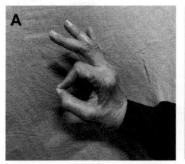
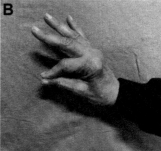

Fig. 2. Demonstration of clinical findings in anterior interosseous nerve syndrome. (*A*) Normal "OK" sign. (*B*) In AION syndrome, weakness of flexor pollicis longus and flexor digitorum profundus would produce a teardrop sign.

Table 1
EDX features of proximal median neuropathies

Site	Nerve Conduction Studies			Needle EMG	
	Median Motor (APB)	Median Sensory (Index)	Thenar Muscles	FPL, PQ, FDP	PT
Ligament of Struthers	ABN	ABN	ABN	ABN	ABN
PT	ABN	ABN	ABN	ABN	Normal
Anterior interosseous nerve syndrome	Normal	Normal	Normal	ABN	Normal

Abbreviations: ABN, abnormal; APB, abductor pollicis brevis; FDP, flexor digitorum profundus digits 2/3; FPL, flexor pollicis longus; PQ, pronator quadratus.

or lumbricals may demonstrate low compound muscle action potential (CMAP) amplitudes. When focal demyelination in the proximal nerve is present, conduction block (CB) or abnormal temporal dispersion may be present in the forearm[2] (**Fig. 3**). If entrapment at the ligament of Struthers is suspected, stimulation can also be performed in the axilla. Although less commonly performed, median motor nerve conduction study recording from the flexor pollicis longus can be performed and reference values have been established.[10] Median F waves may be prolonged in proximal median neuropathies, but these are nonspecific and nonlocalizing.

The median antidromic sensory nerve conduction study is a technically reliable sensory study to assess the median nerve. Recording is routinely made from the index finger, but can be performed from the most symptomatic digit, and a comparison with the unaffected side is important to assess for a relative amplitude reduction, particularly in milder cases. In proximal lesions, the distal latencies are not usually significantly prolonged, although mild prolongation can occur secondary to axonal loss.

Because focal CB is uncommon and nerve conduction studies alone may not precisely localize the site of injury along the nerve, needle electromyography (EMG) may

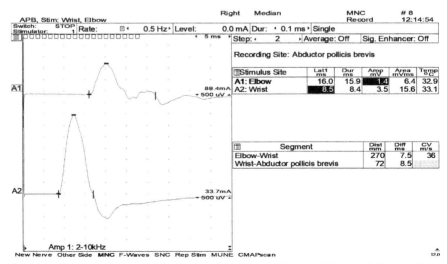

Fig. 3. Median motor nerve conduction study demonstrating partial CB and abnormal temporal dispersion in a proximal median mononeuropathy.

help to more precisely identify localization.[2] The proximal site of injury can often be identified based on the proximal extent of muscles involved. If all muscles, including the PT, are abnormal, the lesion is at or proximal to ligament of Struthers. Muscles supplied by other nerves should also be tested to exclude brachial plexopathy or radiculopathy. The findings on needle EMG reflect the underlying pathophysiology, severity, and chronicity. Fibrillation potentials, reduced recruitment, and long duration motor unit potentials indicate axonal loss and reinnervation. With focal demyelination, decreased recruitment may be the only finding. Specific conditions may demonstrate certain EDX patterns of findings.

Pronator syndrome

In the pronator syndrome, the median nerve is intermittently compressed as it courses through the PT muscle. Rarely, focal demyelination at the site of compression results in CB with abnormal temporal dispersion or slowed conduction velocity between the wrist and the elbow. The median motor distal motor latency (DML) is normal, but the median minimal F waves latency may be prolonged. The sensory nerve conduction study (SNCS) show decreased sensory nerve action potentials (SNAP) amplitudes and normal latency. When severe, EMG demonstrates abnormalities in nearly all median innervated muscles, although the PT is typically spared, because the branch to the muscle is proximal to the median nerve compression as it courses through the muscle. Needle EMG may be normal when only intermittent compression occurs.

Anterior Interosseous syndrome

In AION syndrome, the routine median motor nerve conduction study (MNCS) and SNCS are normal. The median motor nerve conduction study recorded from the pronator quadratus muscle may demonstrate a low CMAP amplitude relative to the unaffected side[11,12] (**Fig. 4**). EMG demonstrates abnormalities in the PQ, FPL, and FDP (digits II and III). In addition to EDX testing, neuromuscular ultrasound examination may be a complementary test to help to confirm a proximal median neuropathy. In

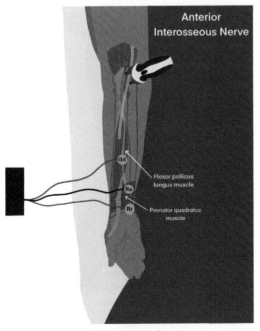

Fig. 4. Anterior interosseous nerve conduction study setup.

a small study of 5 patients with AION syndrome, ultrasound examination demonstrated focal swelling with an hourglass-like constriction of nerve fascicles in several patients.[13]

AXILLARY NEUROPATHY

The axillary nerve arises from the posterior cord of the brachial plexus with fibers derived from the C5 and C6 roots.[3] The nerve winds from anterior to posterior around the neck of the humerus, where it may be prone to injury. It passes through the quadrilateral space in company with the posterior humeral circumflex artery and then divides into anterior, posterior, and collateral branches (**Fig. 5**). The anterior branch provides motor innervation to the deltoid and gives off cutaneous branches that supply the skin overlying the deltoid. The posterior branch supplies the teres minor (TM) and posterior deltoid muscles, and the superior lateral cutaneous nerve supplies the skin over the inferior posterior deltoid and the skin over the long head of the triceps brachii (TB). The collateral branch supplies the long head of the TB muscle.

Etiologies and Clinical Features

Axillary neuropathies most often occur from trauma, including traction at the shoulder, blunt trauma to the shoulder region, dislocation of the humerus at the scapula, or fracture of the surgical neck of the humerus.[14–16] The quadrilateral space syndrome is an uncommon entrapment neuropathy that occurs when the axillary nerve and the posterior humeral circumflex artery become trapped in the quadrilateral space by fibrous tissue accumulation, muscular hypertrophy, tumor, or hematoma.[17,18]

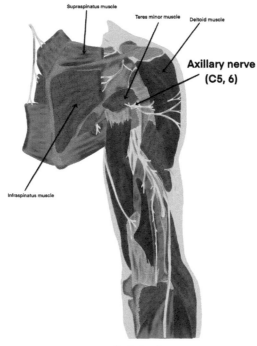

Supraspinatus muscle

Teres minor muscle   Deltoid muscle

Axillary nerve (C5, 6)

Infraspinatus muscle

Posterior view

Fig. 5. Axillary nerve anatomy.

Axillary neuropathy usually manifests with pain or numbness on the lateral arm and weakness of arm abduction beyond 15°. The initial vague symptoms of shoulder pain and weakness can be misdiagnosed as a primary musculoskeletal problem.[14] The quadrilateral space syndrome may be suggested by point tenderness in the posterior quadrilateral space and pain exacerbated by shoulder flexion, abduction, or external rotation.[17]

Electrophysiologic Features

EDX testing can help to confirm an axillary neuropathy and exclude an upper trunk brachial plexopathy or C5 and C6 radiculopathy[14–19] (**Table 2**). The only expected abnormal MNCS is the axillary motor nerve conduction study recording from the deltoid (**Fig. 6**). Because reference values are not well-defined, a greater than 50% decrease in the CMAP amplitude compared with the contralateral side is generally considered abnormal. Although there is no SNCS that test the axillary nerve, other sensory nerve conduction studies (eg, radial or lateral antebrachial cutaneous) are helpful to exclude radial nerve or brachial plexus lesions.

Needle EMG demonstrates abnormalities in the deltoid,TM, or both. Examination of all 3 heads of the deltoid may be useful, because certain fascicles or branches of the axillary nerve may be more affected than others. Additionally, other C5 and C6, non-axillary muscles should be examined. Needle EMG will characterize severity and chronicity of the nerve injury and may include fibrillation potentials, decreased recruitment, and/or long duration motor unit potential.[14,19] There are no published series of EDX findings in patients with axillary mononeuropathies; therefore, the sensitivity of identifying abnormalities on axillary motor nerve conduction study or on needle EMG of individual muscles is unknown.

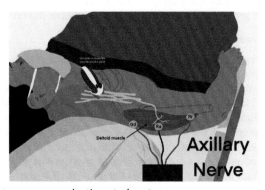

Fig. 6. Axillary motor nerve conduction study setup.

MUSCULOCUTANEOUS NEUROPATHY

The musculocutaneous nerve arises from the termination of the lateral cord of the brachial plexus and consists of fibers derived from the C5 to C7 roots.[3] It courses through the anterior arm, giving off branches to the coracobrachialis, brachialis, and biceps brachii (BB) muscles (**Fig. 7**). It terminates about 2 cm above the elbow as the lateral antebrachial cutaneous nerve, innervating the skin of the lateral cubital and lateral forearm regions.

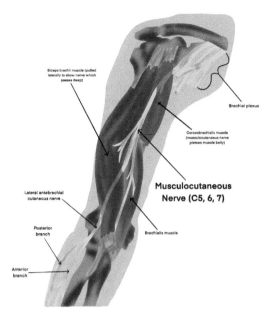

Biceps brachii muscle (pulled laterally to show nerve which passes deep)

Brachial plexus

Coracobrachialis muscle (musculocutaneous nerve pierces muscle belly)

Lateral antebrachial cutaneous nerve

Musculocutaneous Nerve (C5, 6, 7)

Posterior branch

Brachialis muscle

Anterior branch

Fig. 7. Musculocutaneous nerve anatomy.

Etiology and Clinical Features

Causes of musculocutaneous mononeuropathies include traumatic injury, strenuous physical activity or exercise, external compression from casting, trauma to the arm or axillary region, surgery, compression by tumor or hematoma, or involvement from inflammatory conditions (eg, Parsonage Turner syndrome).[20–23] Patients present with weakness involving elbow flexion and possibly mild weakness of elbow supination or arm flexion.[20] Sensory symptoms, when present, involve the lateral cubital and forearm regions and may be reproducible with flexion of the arm against resistance. If the lesion is near the coracoid process, Tinel's sign may be present at the coracoid process.

Electrophysiologic Features

EDX studies can help to confirm a musculocutaneous neuropathy, exclude other mimickers, and determine the severity and degree of recovery[20,22] (see **Table 2**) (**Fig. 8**). Although most injuries produce axonal loss and low musculocutaneous CMAP amplitudes, focal demyelination with CB or abnormal dispersion may occasionally be seen. In a review of 32 patients with musculocutaneous neuropathy or isolated lateral antebrachial cutaneous neuropathy, the musculocutaneous CMAP amplitude and lateral antebrachial SNAP amplitudes were low or absent in the majority, but were normal in some.[24]

In musculocutaneous mononeuropathy, EMG abnormalities are present in the BB and brachialis, without involvement of other C5 and C6 UE muscles. The coracobrachialis muscle is more difficult to examine, but may also show abnormalities.

SUPRASCAPULAR NEUROPATHY

The suprascapular nerve arises from the upper trunk of the brachial plexus and is formed by the ventral rami of C5 and C6.[3] It runs along the superior border of the scapula to the suprascapular notch just below the superior transverse scapular ligament, entering the supraspinous fossa of the posterior scapula giving off branches to the supraspinatus muscle. It passes under the supraspinatus, curves near the lateral border of the scapular spine, and through the spinoglenoid notch to enter the infraspinous fossa of the scapula, giving branches to the infraspinatus muscle (**Fig. 9**). It supplies sensation to the acromioclavicular and glenohumeral joints.

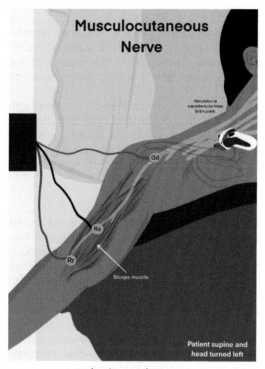

Fig. 8. Musculocutaneous nerve conduction study setup.

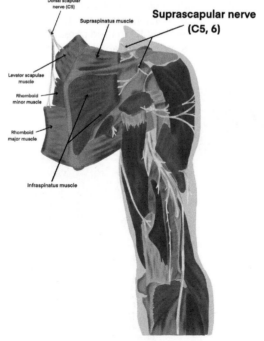

Posterior view

Fig. 9. Suprascapular nerve anatomy.

Etiology and Clinical Features

Suprascapular neuropathies are rare.[25] Etiologies include repetitive overhead activities (occupational or recreational), sports (such as volleyball, pitching in baseball, tennis, swimming, or weight-lifting), traction owing to a rotator cuff tear, direct trauma, or compression from a mass lesion at the suprascapular notch or the spinoglenoid notch.[25–28]

Patients with suprascapular neuropathies present with vague symptoms of shoulder pain and weakness of first 15° of shoulder abduction and external rotation of the humerus. Atrophy of the supraspinatus and infraspinatus muscles may be present on examination.[25] Because patients with rotator cuff disease may present with similar symptoms and signs, EDX testing provides important information about the integrity of the nerve.

Electrophysiologic Features

The EDX abnormalities in suprascapular neuropathies are limited to suprascapular nerve conduction studies and needle EMG abnormalities in the infraspinatus and supraspinatus muscles[26] (**Fig. 10**) (see **Table 2**). The suprascapular motor nerve conduction study, recording from the supraspinatus and/or infraspinatus, shows variable CMAP amplitude reduction. A side-to-side CMAP amplitude difference of 50% or greater is considered abnormal (**Fig. 11**). In a study that included 57 patients with isolated suprascapular neuropathies, the CMAP amplitude did not predict recovery, because there was no significant amplitude difference in patients with and without recovery.[29] Although there are no SNCS to test the suprascapular nerve, other SNCS in the UE are important to exclude an upper trunk brachial plexopathy.

On needle EMG, abnormalities isolated to the supraspinatus and/or infraspinatus, in the absence of abnormalities in other C5 and C6 muscles, confirm a suprascapular neuropathy.[26] Abnormality of both muscles indicates a lesion at the suprascapular notch, whereas abnormality of the infraspinatus alone suggests localization to the spinoglenoid notch. The ability of needle EMG to predict recovery is limited.[29] However, in a small study of 9 patients with paralabral cysts causing a suprascapular

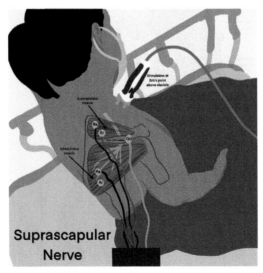

Fig. 10. Suprascapular nerve conduction study setup.

Table 2
EDX features of axillary, musculocutaneous, and suprascapular mononeuropathies compared with C5and C6 radiculopathies and upper trunk brachial plexopathy

Site	Nerve Conduction Studies				Needle EMG			
	Axillary Motor	Musculocutaneous Motor	Suprascapular Motor	LAC	Deltoid/ Teres Minor	Biceps	Supraspinatus and Infraspinatus	Paraspinals
Axillary nerve	ABN	Normal	Normal	Normal	ABN	ABN	Normal	Normal
Musculocutaneous nerve	Normal	ABN	Normal	ABN	Normal	Normal	Normal	Normal
Suprascapular nerve	Normal	Normal	ABN	Normal	Normal	Normal	ABN	Normal
Upper trunk brachial plexus	ABN	ABN	ABN	ABN	ABN	ABN	ABN	Normal
C5-6 Root	ABN	ABN	ABN	Normal	ABN	ABN	ABN	ABN

Abbreviations: ABN, abnormal; LAC, lateral antebrachial cutaneous sensory study.

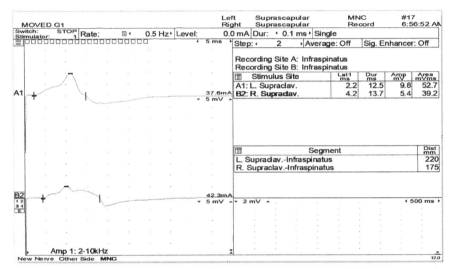

Fig. 11. Suprascapular motor nerve conduction study in a patient with a right suprascapular mononeuropathy. The CMAP is 9.8 on the left (*top trace*) and 5.4 on the right (*bottom trace*).

neuropathy, all patients demonstrated recovery by EMG after decompressive surgery.[30] Furthermore, in some patients with suprascapular mononeuropathy, needle EMG may identify abnormalities indicating a concomitant axillary mononeuropathy, particularly in traumatic cases.[29]

FEMORAL NEUROPATHY

The femoral nerve is the largest branch of the lumbar plexus and is comprised of L2 to L4 nerve roots.[3] The nerve enters Scarpa's triangle after passing beneath the inguinal ligament, lateral to the femoral artery. In the anterior thigh, it travels in a groove between the iliacus and psoas major muscles, outside of the femoral sheath and lateral to the femoral artery. In the thigh, it divides into the anterior and posterior divisions. The anterior division gives off branch to the sartorius muscle and intermediate and medial femoral cutaneous nerves. The posterior division gives off motor branches to the quadriceps (rectus femoris, vastus medialis, vastus intermedius, and vastus lateralis) articularus genus muscles, and saphenous sensory nerve (**Fig. 12**).

Etiologies and Clinical Features

The femoral nerve can be injured from trauma, surgery (abdominal, pelvic, orthopedic), after femoral nerve block or femoral artery puncture, tumor or hematoma (in the abdomen, pelvis, or anterior thigh), compression from abdominal aortic aneurysm, or diabetes.[31–35] Entrapment most commonly occurs under the iliopsoas tendon, the inguinal ligament, or at the adductor canal.[36] Femoral neuropathy presents with variable weakness of hip flexion and knee extension and sensory symptoms in the anterior and medial thigh and anteromedial leg.[31]

Electrophysiologic Features

EDX studies are important to confirm a femoral mononeuropathy and distinguish it from a lumbar (L2–L4) radiculopathy or plexopathy[37] (**Table 3**). A femoral MNCS

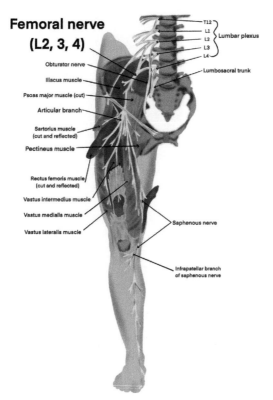

Fig. 12. Femoral nerve anatomy.

(recording from the rectus femoris or vastus medialis) can be technically difficult owing to the deep location of the nerve during stimulation (**Fig. 13**). Side-to-side comparisons to assess for a 50% or greater decrease in the CMAP amplitude is necessary. The saphenous SNCS is the only testable sensory branch of the femoral nerve, but is also a technically difficult nerve conduction studies. Therefore, the diagnosis often relies on needle EMG. On needle EMG, femoral muscles and nonfemoral (eg, obturator innervated) L2 to L4 muscles should be examined to exclude lumbar radiculopathy.[37] The findings in the iliopsoas and quadriceps muscles can localize the lesion in relation to the inguinal ligament.

Table 3
EDX features of obturator and femoral mononeuropathies, L2 and L3 radiculopathies, and lumbar plexopathy

	Nerve Conduction Studies		Needle EMG			
Site	Femoral Motor	Saphenous Sensory	Iliopsoas	Quadriceps	Adductor Longus	Paraspinals
Obturator nerve	Normal	Normal	Normal	Normal	ABN	Normal
Femoral nerve	ABN	ABN	ABN	ABN	Normal	Normal
Lumbar plexus	ABN	ABN	ABN	ABN	ABN	Normal
L2–L3 root	ABN	Normal	ABN	ABN	ABN	ABN

Abbreviations: ABN, abnormal; LAC, lateral antebrachial cutaneous sensory study.

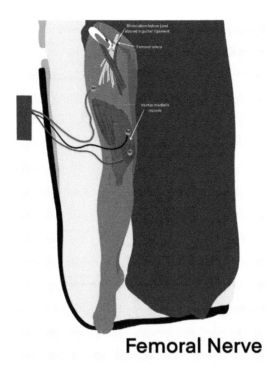

Femoral Nerve

Fig. 13. Femoral motor nerve conduction study setup.

OBTURATOR NEUROPATHY

The obturator nerve arises from the lumbar plexus and is derived from the L2 to L4 roots.[3] It passes through the fibers of the psoas major muscles, emerging at the medial border near the brim of the pelvis. It passes near the common iliac arteries, then along the lateral wall of the lesser pelvis, superior and anterior to the obturator vessels to the upper portion of the obturator foramen. It enters the thigh via the obturator canal and divides into anterior and posterior branches, giving branches to the adductor muscles; external obturator, adductor longus, adductor brevis, adductor magnus, gracilis, and variably to the pectineus muscle. The nerve provides sensory innervation to the medial thigh (**Fig. 14**).

Etiologies and Clinical Features

The obturator nerve may be injured from direct trauma, pelvic surgery, obstetric delivery (particularly with forceps use), tumor or hematoma, entrapment at the obturator canal, or entrapment at the adductor muscle fascia.[36,38–42] Obturator neuropathies often presents with vague symptoms of pain and dysesthesias in the medial thigh or groin.[38–40] Weakness of leg adduction may not be noticed by the patient. When entrapped at the adductor muscle fascia, abduction of the thigh may exacerbate pain and other sensory symptoms.

Electrophysiologic Features

Obturator neuropathy can be confirmed by needle EMG, but there are no reliable nerve conduction studies to study the nerve. Needle EMG will demonstrate

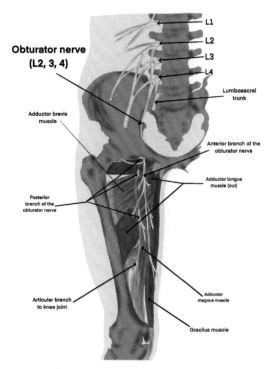

Obturator nerve (L2, 3, 4)

L1
L2
L3
L4

Lumbosacral trunk

Adductor brevis muscle

Anterior branch of the obturator nerve

Adductor longus muscle (cut)

Posterior branch of the obturator nerve

Articular branch to knee joint

Adductor magnus muscle

Gracilus muscle

Fig. 14. Obturator nerve anatomy.

abnormalities in the adductor longus and magnus, but not L2 to L4 muscles supplied by the femoral nerve[39] (see **Table 3**). EDX testing is important to obtain precise localization; in one study, 39% of patients who were referred for a suspected obturator neuropathy were found to have a different disorder.[40]

SCIATIC NEUROPATHY

The sciatic nerve arises from the lower portion of the lumbosacral plexus (with L4–L5, S1–S3 root innervation).[3] It originates in front of the piriformis muscle, passes through the muscle, and courses through the greater sciatic foramen to exit the pelvis (**Fig. 15**). It travels inferiorly in the posterior compartment of the thigh superficial to the adductor magnus muscle to the popliteal fossa, where it divides into the common fibular (peroneal) and the tibial nerves. It gives off motor branches to the hamstrings (biceps femoris, semitendinosus, and semimembranosus) and the adductor magnus. It provides sensory innervation to the skin over the buttocks and posterior thigh, and to the lower leg and foot (except for the anteromedial ankle) through its terminal branches.

Etiology and Clinical Features

Pain in the sciatic nerve distribution is commonly referred to as "sciatica," but this term encompasses many localizations, including lumbosacral radiculopathy. Although sciatica is common and affects between approximately 1% and 40% of people at some point in their life, direct injury or involvement of the sciatic nerve is rare.[43] Etiologies of sciatic neuropathy include direct trauma (eg, penetrating trauma of the buttock or posterior thigh), femur fracture, after gluteal intramuscular injections, hip

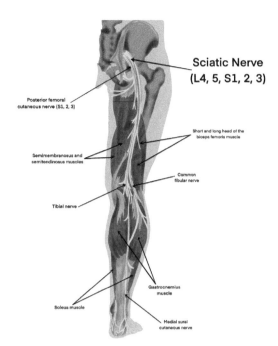

Fig. 15. Sciatic nerve anatomy.

dislocation, hip surgery (eg, hip replacement), and hardware degradation and disintegration within the hip. It can also present during cesarean section or vaginal delivery owing to positioning (greater thigh flexion is associated with a greater risk for sciatic nerve traction), or compression by a tumor or hematoma.[44–51] In a recent study of 109 patients from a single institution with sciatic neuropathy from nonpenetrating trauma, 56% were related to LE injury such as hip replacement, 15% related to compression, and a small percentage related to inflammation, radiation, ischemia, or other causes.[52] The sciatic nerve may also rarely be entrapped as it courses through the piriformis muscle, resulting in piriformis syndrome.[50] Piriformis syndrome may result from an overuse injury, anatomic variation, piriformis muscle spasms, or by pseudoaneurysm of the inferior gluteal artery.[51,53,54]

Sciatic neuropathy often presents with nonspecific painful sensory symptoms and weakness.[45,55] Sensory features consist of pain overlying the ipsilateral buttock and posterior thigh, as well as numbness or paresthesia. Some weakness of knee flexion may also occur. More complete or severe sciatic neuropathy may present with weakness and sensory disturbance involving the foot as well as the hamstring region, which can mimic fibular (peroneal) and tibial mononeuropathies. In sciatic neuropathy, peroneal fibers are more susceptible to stretch injury than tibial fibers. Sensory features may involve the entire foot and leg, except the anteromedial ankle (saphenous distribution). Piriformis syndrome typically presents as pain in the buttock or hip area, radiating pain or numbness that can extend into the calf, nonspecific weakness that can affect part or all of the leg, ankle, and foot owing to involvement of peroneal and tibial fibers.[51,53,54]

Electrophysiologic Features

Given the clinical similarities of sciatic neuropathy and lumbosacral radiculopathy, EDX is useful to assist in localization, as well as determine the chronicity and severity of the injury[52,55,56] (**Table 4**). Abnormalities in the peroneal, tibial, or both MNCS are typical (**Fig. 16**A, B). The sural and superficial peroneal SNAP and the peroneal motor study recording from the extensor digitorum brevis (EDB) have been shown to be more sensitive compared with the tibial motor study; only 60% of patients had abnormalities in both peroneal and tibial CMAPs and sural and superficial peroneal sensory nerve action potentials.[52] F waves and H reflexes may be prolonged or absent, but these are nonspecific and nonlocalizing, because they can also be abnormal in radiculopathies and plexopathies.[57] H reflex latency may show changes with provocative tests in piriformis syndrome.[54] Abnormal SNAP responses help to distinguish sciatic neuropathy, in which the superficial peroneal, sural, and/or plantar responses are abnormal, from a lumbosacral radiculopathy (in which SNAP are normal). However, abnormal sensory nerve action potentials can also occur with lumbosacral plexus localization. Because low motor and sensory nerve conduction studies amplitudes may also be seen in a polyneuropathy, side-to-side comparison is important when a sciatic neuropathy is suspected.

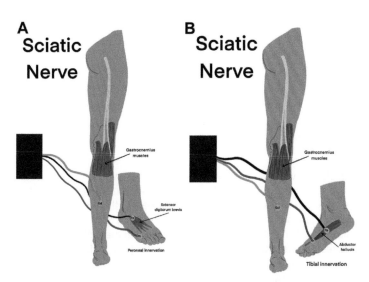

Fig. 16. Nerve conduction studies to test the motor branches of the sciatic nerve. (*A*) Recording from the extensor digitorum brevis muscle. (*B*) Recording from the abductor hallucis.

Needle EMG demonstrates abnormalities to a variable degree in muscles supplied by the peroneal and tibial nerves in the lower leg, biceps femoris, but sparing muscles supplied by the superior and inferior gluteal innervated muscle (eg, gluteus medius or tensor fasciae latae, and gluteus maximus) muscles in the lower leg have been shown to be abnormal more frequently than hamstring muscles, with abnormalities in the hamstring muscles being present approximately 45% of the time.[52] Abnormalities are more coming in peroneal-innervated muscles in nearly all patients with sciatic neuropathies but in tibial-innervated muscles in 74% to 84% of patients.[56]

TIBIAL NEUROPATHY

The tibial nerve arises from the sciatic nerve in the popliteal fossa.[3] It courses through the popliteal fossa giving off branches to the gastrocnemii, soleus, plantaris, and

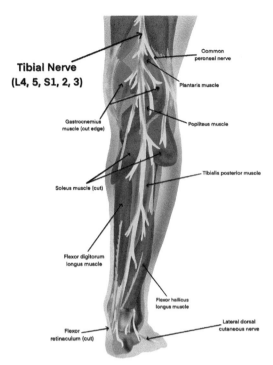

Fig. 17. Tibial nerve anatomy.

popliteus muscles as well as sensory branches to the lower one-half of the posterior leg and the lateral border of the foot to the tip of the fifth toe (**Fig. 17**). At the inferior border of the popliteal fossa, the nerve courses deep to the tendinous arch of the soleus and enters the posterior leg. It continues inferiorly and medially, reaching the posteromedial aspect of the ankle between the medial malleolus and the calcaneus. In the leg, it gives off branches to the tibialis posterior (TP), FDL, flexor hallucis longus, and deep portion of the soleus. It terminates deep in the flexor retinaculum, dividing into the medial and lateral plantar and medial and lateral calcaneal nerves (**Fig. 18**). The medial and lateral plantar nerves supply the skin of the medial and lateral sole, respectively, and provide innervation to many of the intrinsic foot muscles (**Fig. 19**).

Etiology and Clinical Features

Etiologies of tibial neuropathies include direct trauma, ischemia, and masses (eg, Baker's cyst, tumor, or hematoma). Tarsal tunnel syndrome (TTS) is a rare tibial entrapment neuropathy at the flexor retinaculum at the ankle, and may result from osseous compression (owing to bone spurs, fracture fragments, tarsal coalition), mass lesions (ganglia, nerve sheath tumors, fibrous tissue, hypertrophic muscles, accessory muscles), congenital foot deformities, or systemic diseases (diabetes, vasculitis, rarely uremia).[58–61]

Proximal tibial mononeuropathies at the popliteal fossa or leg have variable presentations.[58] Lesions in the popliteal fossa or above the leg present with weakness of ankle plantarflexion, inversion, toe flexion, and sensory deficits in the lower portion of the posterior leg and the lateral side of the foot to the end of the fifth toe, and bottom of the foot. Tarsal tunnel syndrome most commonly presents with foot and ankle pain

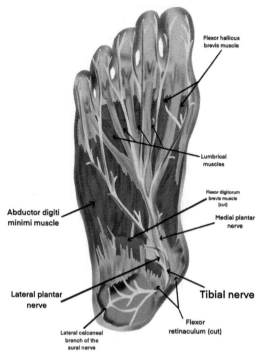

Fig. 18. Anatomy of the distal branches of the tibial nerve.

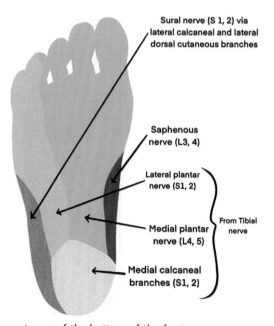

Fig. 19. Sensory dermatomes of the bottom of the foot.

Table 4
EDX features of sciatic and tibial mononeuropathies compared with sacral plexopathy

Site	Nerve Conduction Studies						Needle EMG		
	Peroneal Motor	Tibial Motor	Sural	Medial/Lateral Plantar	Tibial Foot Muscles	Gastrocnemius, Soleus	Anterior Tibialis, Peroneal Foot Muscles	Hamstrings	Gluteus Medius, Gluteus Maximus
Sciatic nerve	ABN	ABN	ABN	ABN	ABN	ABN	ABN	ABN	Normal
Tibial nerve at the knee	Normal	ABN	ABN	ABN	ABN	ABN	Normal	Normal	Normal
Tibial nerve at the ankle	Normal	ABN	Normal	ABN	ABN	Normal	Normal	ABN	Normal
Sacral plexus	ABN	ABN	ABN	ABN	ABN	ABN	ABN	ABN	ABN

Abbreviation: ABN, abnormal.

that is burning in character and exacerbated by weight bearing and worse at night.[58,59] Perimalleolar pain, numbness, and paresthesia, as well as atrophy of intrinsic foot muscles may be present.

Electrophysiologic Features

EDX testing is helpful to confirm the diagnosis and exclude alternative pathologies such as polyneuropathy, S1 radiculopathy, sciatic neuropathy, and lumbosacral plexopathy[62] (see **Table 4**). Tibial motor nerve conduction study can be recorded from the abductor hallucis and abductor digiti minimi pedis (**Fig. 20**). Transtarsal medial and lateral plantar mixed nerve conduction studies will often demonstrate low amplitudes, and the sural amplitude may be variably affected because the sural is composed of branches form the fibular/peroneal and tibial nerves.

Needle EMG demonstrates abnormalities in tibial innervated foot muscles at any site of injury to the tibial nerve, but abnormalities in these muscles are difficult to interpret in older individuals. More proximal muscles, such as the gastrocnemii and TP help to determine the proximal extent of the injury. A 2005 American Association of Neuromuscular and Electrodiagnostic Medicine practice parameter reviewed the literature to assess the role of EDX studies in TTS.[62] Although the number of high-quality studies was limited, SNCS and mixed nerve conduction studies abnormalities were present in 85% to 93% of patients with the lateral plantar sensory response more commonly absent than the medial plantar response. Prolonged tibial DML to the AH were only present in 21% to 52% of individuals, indicating that MNCS are less sensitive than sensory nerve conduction studies in the diagnosis of tarsal tunnel syndrome. There

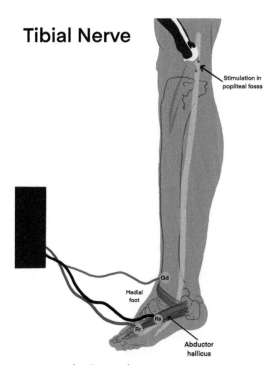

Fig. 20. Tibial motor nerve conduction study setup.

were no studies that directly assessed the utility of needle EMG in the evaluation of TTS. In the presence of significant polyneuropathy, the diagnosis of TTS may be difficult to confirm; prolonged latencies are more common, but low amplitudes can occur.[59,62]

SUMMARY

Electrodiagnosis is an important tool that complements the clinical assessment of patients with suspected uncommon mononeuropathies. Knowledge of the anatomy and understanding the pattern of findings on nerve conduction studies and needle EMG help to diagnoses these conditions and exclude more common mimickers. The EDX often requires technically difficult or less commonly performed studies, making diagnosis more challenging.

CLINICS CARE POINTS

- Detailed knowledge of neuroanatomy is crucial for diagnosis of uncommon neuropathies. Brief neuromuscular examination before the electrodiagnostic study will help to tailor the study and make the correct diagnosis.
- Contralateral studies are usually very helpful to diagnose mild to moderate uncommon neuropathies.
- Detailed electromyography can localize the lesion when the nerves are not easily accessible for conduction studies

ACKNOWLEDGMENTS

Illustrations by Ms Danielle Rinck.

REFERENCES

1. Dang AC, Rodner CM. Unusual compression neuropathies of the forearm, part II: median nerve. J Hand Surg Am 2009;34(10):1915–20.
2. Gross PT, Jones HR. Proximal median neuropathies: electromyographic and clinical correlation. Muscle Nerve 1992;15:390–5.
3. Standring S. Gray's anatomy: the anatomical basis of clinical practice. 41st edition. Elsevier Limited; 2016.
4. Campbell WW, Landau ME. Controversial entrapment neuropathies. Neurosurg Clin N Am 2008;19(4):597–608.
5. Dawson DM, Hallet M, Wilbourn AJ. Entrapment neuropathies. third ed. Philadelphia: Lippincott; 1999.
6. Kumar GR. A study of the incidence of supracondylar process of the humerus. J Anat Soc India 2008;57(2):111–5.
7. Gross PT, Tolomedo EA. Proximal median neuropathies. Neurol Clin 1999;17(3): 425–45.
8. Schantz K, Riegels-Nielsen P. The anterior interosseous nerve syndrome. J Hand Surg 1992;17(5).
9. Pham M, Bäumer P, et al. Anterior interosseous nerve syndrome: fascicular motor lesions of median nerve trunk. Neurology 2014;82(7):598–606.

10. Vuvic S, Yiannikas C. Anterior interosseous nerve conduction study: normative data. Muscle Nerve 2007;35:119–21.

11. Rosenberg JN. Anterior interosseous/median nerve latency ratio. Arch Phys Med Rehabil 1990;71:228–30.

12. Nakano KK, Lundergan C, Okihiro MM. Anterior interosseous nerve syndromes: diagnostic methods and alternative treatments. Arch Neurol 1977;34:477–80.

13. Noda Y, Sekiguchi K, Tokuoka H, et al. Ultrasonographic findings of proximal median neuropathy: a case series of suspected distal neuralgic amyotrophy. J Neurol Sci 2017;377:1–5.

14. Steinmann SP, Moran EA. Axillary nerve injury: diagnosis and treatment. J Am Acad Orthop Surg 2001;9(5):328–35.

15. Davidson LT, Carter GT, et al. Iatrogenic axillary neuropathy after intramuscular injection of the deltoid muscle. Am J Phys Med Rehabil 2007;86(6):507–11.

16. Paladini D, Dellantonio R, et al. Axillary neuropathy in volleyball players: report of two cases and literature review. J Neurol Neurosurg Psychiatry 1996;60:345–7.

17. Cahill BR, Palmer RE. Quadrilateral space syndrome. J Hand Surg 1983; 8(1):65–9.

18. Linker CS, Helms CA, Fritz RC. Quadrilateral space syndrome: findings at MR imaging. Radiology 1993;188(3).

19. De Laat EAT, Visser CPJ, et al. Nerve lesions in primary shoulder dislocations and humeral neck fractures: a prospective clinical and EMG study. J Bone Joint Surg Br 1994;76-B(3):381–3.

20. Beslega D, Castellano V, et al. Musculocutaneous neuropathy: case report and discussion. HSS J 2010;6:112–6.

21. Mastaglia FL. Musculocutaneous neuropathy after strenuous physical activity. Med J Aust 1986;145(3–4):153–4.

22. Yilmaz C, Eskandari MM, Colak M. Traumatic musculocutaneous neuropathy: a case report. Arch Orthop Trauma Surg 2005;125:414–6.

23. Juel VC, Kiely JM, et al. Isolated musculocutaneous neuropathy caused by a proximal humeral exostosis. Neurology 2000;54(2):494.

24. O'Gorman CM, Kassardjian C, Sorenson EJ. Musculocutaneous neuropathy. Muscle Nerve 2018;58:726–9.

25. Boykin RE, Friedman DJ, et al. Suprascapular neuropathy. J Bone Joint Surg 2010;92(13):2348–64.

26. Anthony R, Rotenberg D, Bach BR Jr. Suprascapular neuropathy. J Am Acad Orthop Surg 1999;7(6):358–67.

27. Ferretti A, Cerullo G, Russo G. Suprascapular neuropathy in volleyball players. J Bone Joint Surg 1987;69-A(2):260–3.

28. Ringel SP, Treihaft M, Carr M. Suprascapular neuropathy in pitchers. Am J Sports Med 1990;18(1):80–6.

29. Memon AB, Dymm B, Ahmad BK, et al. Suprascapular neuropathy: a review of 87 cases. Muscle Nerve 2019;60:250–3.

30. Feinberg JH, Mehta P, Gulotta LV, et al. Electrodiagnostic evidence of suprascapular nerve recovery after decompression. Muscle Nerve 2019;59:247–9.

31. Kuntzer T, Mell GV, Regli F. Clinical and prognostic features in unilateral femoral neuropathies. Muscle Nerve 1998;20(2):205–11.

32. Moore AE, Stringer MD. Iatrogenic femoral nerve injury: a systematic review. Surg Radiol Anat 2011;33:649–58.

33. Coppack SW, Watkins PJ. The natural history of diabetic femoral neuropathy. Q J Med 1991;79(1):307–13.

34. Rosenblum J, Schwarz GA, Bendler E. Femoral neuropathy - a neurological complication of hysterectomy. JAMA 1966;195(6):409–14.
35. Merchant RF, Cafferata HT, DePalma RG. Ruptured aortic aneurysm seen initially as acute femoral neuropathy. Arch Surg 1982;117(6):811–3.
36. Martin R, Martin HD, Kivlan BR. Nerve entrapment in the hip region: current concepts review. Int J Sports Phys Ther 2017;12(7):1163–73.
37. Jillapalli D, Shefner JM. Electrodiagnosis in common mononeuropathies and plexopathies. Semin Neurol 2005;25(2):196–203.
38. Craig A. Entrapment neuropathies of the lower extremity. PM R 2013;5(5 suppl): S31–40.
39. Tipton JS. Obturator neuropathy. Curr Rev Musculoskelet Med 2008;1:234–7.
40. Sorenson EJ, Chen JJ, Daube JR. Obturator neuropathy: causes and outcome. Muscle Nerve 2002;25(4):605–7.
41. Harvey G, Bell S. Obturator neuropathy: an anatomic perspective. Clin Orthop Relat Res 1999;363:203–11.
42. Warfield CA. Obturator neuropathy after forceps delivery. Obstet Gynecol 1984; 64(3 suppl):47S–8S.
43. Cook CE, Taylor J, et al. Risk factors for the first time incidence sciatica: a systematic review. Physiother Res Int 2013;19(2):65–78.
44. Valat J-P, Genevay S, et al. Sciatica. Best Pract Res Clin Rheumatol 2010;24(2): 241–52.
45. Yuen EC, So YT. Sciatic neuropathy. Neurol Clin 1999;17(3):617–31.
46. Roy S, Levine AB, et al. Intraoperative positioning during Cesarean as a cause of sciatic neuropathy. Obstet Gynecol 2002;99(4):652–3.
47. McQuarrie HG, Harris JW, et al. Sciatic neuropathy complicating vaginal hysterectomy. Am J Obstet Gynecol 1972;113(2):223–32.
48. Fleming RE Jr, Michelsen CB. Sciatic paralysis: a complication of bleeding following hip surgery. J Bone Joint Surg 1979;61-A(1):37–9.
49. Plewnia C, Wallace C, Zochodne D. Traumatic sciatic neuropathy: a novel cause, local experience, and a review of the literature. J Trauma Acute Care Surg 1999; 47(5):986.
50. Parziale JR, Hudgins TH, Fishman LM. The piriformis syndrome. Am J Orthop (Belle Mead NJ) 1996;25(12):819–23.
51. Papadopoulos SM, McGillicuddy JE, Albers JW. Unusual cause of "piriformis muscle syndrome." Arch Neurol 1990;47:1144–6.
52. Cherian RP, Li Y. Clinical and electrodiagnostic features of nontraumatic sciatic neuropathy. Muscle Nerve 2019;59(3):309–14.
53. Papadopoulos SM, McGillicuddy JE, Messina LM. Pseudoaneurysm of the inferior gluteal artery presenting as sciatic nerve compression. Neurosurgery 1989; 24:926–8.
54. Fishman LM, Zybert PA. Electrophysiologic evidence of piriformis syndrome. Arch Phys Med Rehabil 1992;73:359–64.
55. Yuen EC, Olney RK, So YT. Sciatic neuropathy: clinical and prognostic features in 73 patients. Neurology 1994;44(9):1669.
56. Yuen EC, So YT, Olney RK. The electrophysiologic features of sciatic neuropathy in 100 patients. Muscle Nerve 1995;18(4):414–20.
57. Goodgold J. H reflex. Arch Phys Med Rehabil 1976;57:407.
58. Drees C, Wilbourn AJ, Stevens HGJ. Main trunk tibial neuropathies. Neurology 2002;59(7):1082–4.
59. Oh SJ, Meyer RD. Entrapment neuropathies of the tibial (posterior tibial) nerve. Neurol Clin 1999;17(3):593–615.

60. Lee J-H, Jun J-B, et al. Posterior tibial neuropathy by a Baker's cyst: case report. Korean J Intern Med 2000;15(1):96–8.
61. Dimberg EL, Rubin DI, et al. Popliteus muscle hemorrhage as a rare cause of proximal tibial neuropathy. J Clin Neurosci 2014;21(3):520–1.
62. Patel AT, Gaines K, et al. Usefulness of electrodiagnostic techniques in the evaluation of suspected tarsal tunnel syndrome: an evidence-based review. Muscle Nerve 2005;32:236–40.

Electrodiagnostic Assessment of Radiculopathies

Robert J. Marquardt, DO, Kerry H. Levin, MD*

KEYWORDS

- Radiculopathy • Electromyography • Electrodiagnosis • Neuromuscular

KEY POINTS

- Nerve conduction studies are limited in their utility to diagnose radiculopathy. They should be used primarily to exclude alternative diagnoses.
- A needle examination root screen approach should include a minimum of 6 muscles covering all common root levels.
- On needle electrode examination, spontaneous activity and/or motor unit action potential morphologic changes in 2 different muscles of the same myotome, but with different peripheral nerve innervation, supports an electrodiagnosis of motor radiculopathy.

INTRODUCTION

One of the most common referrals to the electrodiagnostic laboratory is for evaluation of clinically suspected radiculopathy, a pathologic process involving the nerve root. In 1950, Shea and colleagues[1] first described how electrodiagnosis (EDX) could identify fibrillation potentials in a specific myotome, thereby supporting a diagnosis of compressive radiculopathy. Despite being a common referral indication, EDX confirmation of a radiculopathy is challenging due to several limitations of testing. A study of 1000 patients referred for electromyography (EMG) evaluation of radiculopathy found 49.8% with a normal study and only 7% confirming radiculopathy.[2] Sensory symptoms and pain are the most common complaints,[3] but because small unmyelinated pain fibers or preganglionic sensory fibers cannot be assessed by routine nerve conduction studies (NCSs), patients often have a normal study even if the pathology truly involves the root. Despite the limitations of EDX testing in the diagnosis of radiculopathy, EMG plays an important role. When EMG is combined with a clinical history, examination, and other testing, it can support the diagnosis of radiculopathy and exclude mimicking disorders.[4]

Neuromuscular Center, Department of Neurology, Cleveland Clinic, 9500 Euclid Avenue, Desk S90, Cleveland, OH 44195, USA
* Corresponding author.
E-mail address: levink@ccf.org

Neurol Clin 39 (2021) 983–995
https://doi.org/10.1016/j.ncl.2021.06.011
neurologic.theclinics.com

REVIEW OF ANATOMY

There are 31 nerve root pairs: 8 cervical, 12 thoracic, 5 lumbar, 5 sacral, and 1 coccygeal. Each root is formed from a ventral motor axon whose cell body originates in the anterior horn cell of the ventral spinal cord and a dorsal sensory axon whose cell body originates from the dorsal root ganglion (DRG). The DRG typically is located along the dorsal root at the entrance of the intervertebral foramen, and thus is not truly intraspinal. Approximately 3% to 9% of L3 and L4 DRGs, 11% to 38% of L5 DRGs, and 71% to 77% of S1 DRGs are intraspinal.[5–7] Similarly, in the cervical region, there has been suggestion that the C5 and C6 DRGs can be intraspinal.[8]

The ventral motor and postganglionic dorsal sensory axons come together within the central canal to form the nerve root, which then exits the canal via the intervertebral foramen (**Fig. 1**). Upon exiting laterally from the intervertebral foramen, the nerve root divides into small posterior primary ramus, supplying the neck and paraspinal muscles, and a larger anterior primary ramus supplies the limbs and anterior trunk, including the abdominal and intercostal muscles.

From C1 to C7, the nerve root exits above the corresponding vertebral body (eg, the C7 root exits from the C6-7 intervertebral foramen). The C8 nerve root is a transition point and exits between the C7 and T1 vertebral bodies and all subsequent roots exit below their corresponding vertebral body. The cervical, thoracic, and high lumbar segments the root exit laterally essentially along a horizontal plane. Because the spinal cord ends in the adult at approximately the L2 vertebral body, however, the nerve roots representing segments below this level must travel caudally within the central canal to reach their exiting intervertebral foramen. This collective group of nerve roots forms the cauda equina. Because they travel together, pathology at the L3 level

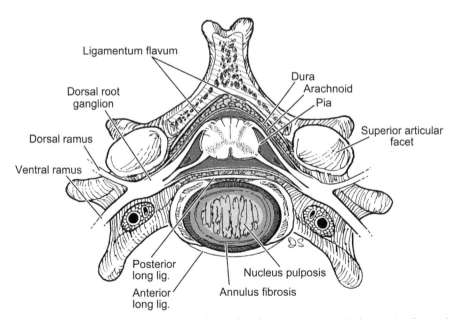

Fig. 1. Anatomy of the spine. The ventral and dorsal roots are intraspinal, meaning located within the central canal. The dorsal root ganglion is located at the entrance of the intervertebral foramen, and thus is not truly intraspinal. long, longitudinal; lig, ligament. (*Reprinted with permission*, Cleveland Clinic Center for Medical Art & Photography ©2021. All Rights Reserved).

potentially could have an impact on not only the L3 nerve root but also the descending nerve roots traveling as part of the cauda equina.

Almost all muscles receive innervation from more than 1 nerve root, and the degree to which each nerve root segment contributes innervation is unpredictable and can vary among individuals.[9]

NERVE CONDUCTION STUDIES

An EDX study evaluating for potential radiculopathy starts with NCSs. Nerves selected for testing are guided by clinical history, examination, and the requisition from the ordering provider. Commonly used NCSs are listed in **Table 1** for the upper limb and **Table 2** for the lower limb. Normative values based on age, gender, and height have been published.[10,11]

Several factors limit the utility of NCSs in the diagnosis of radiculopathy. Disc protrusion and spondylosis are among the most common causes of compressive radiculopathy but often result in damage to only a small number of traversing nerve fibers, producing limited motor and sensory symptoms. Paresthesias and pain, which often are the predominant complaints in radiculopathy, are transmitted via unmyelinated C-type sensory fibers that are not evaluated using routine NCS techniques. Furthermore, focal compression of a nerve root could cause focal conduction velocity slowing and/or conduction block along the compressed segment. These are not identifiable, however, because intraspinal location of most radicular lesions render direct NCSs on the nerve root proximal to the compressed area impossible.

Sensory Nerve Conduction Studies

Sensory NCSs are of limited value in the diagnosis of radiculopathy. The sensory nerve action potential (SNAP) responses are not affected in radiculopathy because most radicular lesions are located within the central canal and proximal neural foramen.

Table 1		
Common nerve conduction studies performed in the upper limb		
Nerve	Recording Site	Root Distribution
Sensory conduction responses		
Median	Digit 1	C6
	Digit 2	C6-7
	Digit 3	C7
Ulnar	Digit 4–5	C8 (T1)
Radial	Dorsal hand	C6 (7)
LAC	Forearm	C6
MAC	Forearm	T1
Motor conduction responses		
Median	APB	(C8) T1
Ulnar	ADM	C8 (T1)
Radial	EDC	C8
Musculocutaneous	Biceps	C5-6
Axillary	Deltoid	C5-6

Abbreviations: EDC, extensor digitorum communis; LAC, lateral antebrachial cutaneous; MAC, medial antebrachial cutaneous.

Table 2
Common nerve conduction studies performed in the lower limb

Nerve	Recording Site	Root Distribution
Sensory conduction responses		
Sural	Lateral ankle	S1
Superficial peroneal	Dorsum of foot	L5
Saphenous	Medial foreleg	L3-4
Motor conduction responses		
Tibial	Abductor hallucis	S1
Peroneal	EDB	L5 (S1)
Peroneal	Tibialis anterior	(L4) L5
Femoral	Rectus femoris	L3-4

Because most DRGs reside distal to the area of nerve root compression, the SNAPs remain normal. If the lesion is noncompressive (ie, infiltrative) or extraspinal (distal to the neural foramen), the DRG can be damaged leading to wallerian degeneration and SNAP amplitude reduction or loss. Examples of this include malignancy and infection.

One exception is the L5 DRG, which sometimes can reside within the central canal where it is vulnerable to intraspinal compression.[12] This can result in an absent or low amplitude superficial fibular (peroneal) sensory response. The S1 DRG also can reside within the central canal; it typically rests below the L5-S1 disc space where most compressive pathology occurs; thus, the sural SNAP remains unaffected.[13] The value of sensory NCSs primarily is to assess for other lesions, such as mononeuropathy and plexopathy, because their clinical presentation can mimic radiculopathy.[14]

Testing the median, ulnar, and superficial radial SNAPs usually is adequate to screen for common mimics, such as carpal tunnel syndrome, ulnar mononeuropathy, or peripheral neuropathy affecting the arm (see **Table 1**). If a C5-6 root lesion is in question, adding a lateral antebrachial cutaneous SNAP may be appropriate to rule out an upper trunk brachial plexopathy. Similarly, a medial antebrachial cutaneous sensory response could help rule out a lower trunk brachial plexopathy mimicking a T1 radiculopathy.

For patients presenting with a suspected lumbosacral radiculopathy, the superficial fibular and sural nerves are most useful (see **Table 2**). These responses can be obtained reliably in most individuals; although, after the ages of 50 and 75, respectively, their absence may be a normal finding.[15,16] Normal sensory responses help to rule out mimics, such as peripheral neuropathy, peroneal mononeuropathy, sciatic mononeuropathy, and sacral plexopathy. Saphenous and lateral femoral cutaneous SNAPs also can be performed but are technically challenging. Asymmetric amplitude reduction or absence may be useful to exclude a femoral mononeuropathy or lumbar plexopathy mimicking an L3 or L4 root lesion.

Motor Nerve Conduction Studies

Motor NCSs can be useful in radiculopathy assessment but have limitations and frequently are normal.[17] Typically, compressive intraspinal lesions damage a limited number of motor fibers of the traversing nerve root. The recorded compound muscle action potential (CMAP) reflects the summation of all underlying muscle fiber action potentials within the recording electrode field. At least 50% of motor axons must be lost to produce a reliably abnormal CMAP difference compared with the contralateral side.[18] Timing between the onset of the lesion and the study also is important, because the CMAP may not decrease until sufficient time has passed for wallerian degeneration to take place (at least 5 days post-transection). Similarly, reinnervation can result in normalization of previously reduced CMAP amplitudes.

Reliable CMAPs can be obtained from C5-6, C8, and T1 myotomes (see **Table 1**). The median CMAP response recording abductor pollicis brevis (APB) reflects T1 root/segment innervation, whereas the musculocutaneous CMAP recording over biceps and axillary CMAP recording over deltoid reflect the C5-6 roots/segments. In a C8 lesion, the ulnar CMAP recording abductor digiti minimi (ADM) could be reduced, and an amplitude less than 10.2 mV was shown to have sensitivity and specificity of 0.86 and 0.74, respectively, in NEE-confirmed active radiculopathy.[19] The C7 myotome has no reliable CMAP because the muscles are not spatially isolated from muscles of other myotomes.[20]

In the leg, L5 and S1 myotomes are well represented with routine studies (see **Table 2**). The fibular CMAP (recording extensor digitorum brevis [EDB] and tibialis anterior) reflects predominantly the L5 myotome. The tibial CMAP reflects predominantly the S1 myotome. For NEE-confirmed active L5 radiculopathy, a fibular CMAP amplitude less than 3.6 mV was shown to have sensitivity and specificity of 0.92 and 0.60, respectively.[19] Femoral motor NCS recording rectus femoris can show axon loss at the L3 and L4 root levels.

Routine motor NCSs obtained in the arm as part of a screening assessment include the median (recording APB) and the ulnar (recording ADM). These studies, however, evaluate the C8 and T1 roots, which are not the most common levels involved in cervical radiculopathy.[21] In the lower limb, routine motor NCSs obtained include the fibular (EDB) and the tibial response recording abductor hallucis, which assess the commonly involved L5 and S1 root levels.

If an abnormality is noted on NCS, it is good practice to obtain the same response on the contralateral side for comparison. It also is important to note any other technical factors, such as peripheral edema and obesity, which could contribute to spuriously reduced CMAP amplitudes.[22]

LATE RESPONSES

Late responses include both the F wave and H reflex. In radiculopathy, both can be of potential value because the evoked motor potential travels to the spinal cord and back down through the nerve root, theoretically allowing for assessment of the nerve root itself.

F Wave

An F response is a pure motor arc that measures the time it takes for an evoked antidromic motor nerve action potential to travel proximally up the peripheral nerve from the point of stimulation and reactivate a small number of anterior horn cells' axon hillocks, triggering a backfire that sends the action potential orthodromically back down the motor peripheral nerve to the recording electrode. The most common measurement for assessment is the earliest latency. In root compression, the very narrow segment of slowing is diluted by the longer segment of normal conduction, thus reducing sensitivity of the response. Other parameters, such as chronodispersion and persistence, have been studied but are less reliable.[23]

Commonly obtained F responses include the ulnar response (ADM) and median (APB) in the arm and the fibular (EDB) and tibial (abductor hallucis) in the leg, which all are highly reproducible.[24,25] Using the motor CMAP and F response together can be beneficial in interpretation, but studies have concluded F responses have relatively low sensitivity in this regard.[26] In a recent study of 142 patients with unilateral L5 (n = 67) or S1 (n = 76) radiculopathy in whom magnetic resonance imaging and NEE correlated, abnormal fibular and tibial F responses were found only 50.7% and 36.0% of the time, respectively.[23] Because F waves represent a pure motor arc, they are normal in patients with only sensory complaints.

The radial F wave technique (recording form anconeus and extensor indicis proprius) has been validated with normative values published.[27,28] In theory, an F wave can be obtained from any peripheral motor nerve but the clinical utility of other responses is not clear.

H Reflex

The tibial H reflex is a true root reflex arc that involves both the sensory and motor roots and is a highly sensitive measure of S1 root pathology (up to 80% in surgically proved cases).[29] A recent study also suggests that the lateral or medial gastrocnemius also could be recorded without reduced sensitivity.[30]

An abnormal H reflex with a normal tibial CMAP is suggestive of more proximal disease, which could be anywhere along the reflex arc, including the S1 root, sciatic nerve, or proximal tibial nerve; thus, specificity as an isolated abnormality is low. Also, limb length, temperature, and age have an impact on the response. Therefore, a side-to-side comparison of the H amplitude is felt to be of highest clinical utility, with an H-amplitude ratio (abnormal H amplitude divided by contralateral H amplitude) of less than 0.4 being abnormal.[31] The absence of an H reflex on 1 side when present on the other always is abnormal, whereas bilateral absence could be technical in nature, particularly in large individuals. An H amplitude of less than 1 mV or the absence of an H reflex in a person above age 60 is considered a possible normal finding.

NEEDLE ELECTRODE EXAMINATION

The needle electrode examination (NEE) is more valuable than NCSs in the assessment of radiculopathy. The sensitivity of the NEE has been reported to range from 49% to 86% for lumbosacral to 50% to 71% for cervical motor radiculopathies.[32] Specificity has been found to range from 87% to 100%, depending on the abnormalities identified in lumbosacral radiculopathy.[33,34] Specificity was 100% if fibrillations and positive waves (PWs) were seen in 2 limb muscles with or without the corresponding paraspinal muscle, or in 1 limb and its corresponding paraspinal muscle. If greater than 30% polyphasia was utilized as the abnormal finding, the specificity dropped to the lower end of the range. In light of the lag in generation of fibrillation potentials after acute nerve transection, delaying NEE for at least 3 weeks after the onset of motor symptoms is recommended.

One of the reasons for low sensitivity of NEE relates to the need for motor axon loss or significant motor root demyelination to occur for changes to be seen on NEE. If a lesion affects only the sensory root fibers, NEE is normal. Therefore, a normal NEE does not rule out radiculopathy as a cause for the clinical symptoms if sensory symptoms are the main complaint.

The American Association of Neuromuscular & Electrodiagnostic Medicine recommends a root screen approach to the design of the NEE study to ensure that screening of the most common root levels involved in radiculopathy is performed.[35] In the arm, this includes C5-8 and in the leg L3-S1. If an abnormality is found, additional muscles in the same myotome are studied. The more muscles in a myotome showing consistent change, the more reliable the diagnosis. A minimum of 2 muscles in the same myotome with different peripheral nerve innervation is minimum criterion for EDX of motor radiculopathy.[9] Identifying both distal and proximal muscle involvement further supports the diagnosis and rules out peripheral causes like polyneuropathy or mononeuropathy.

Recently, a 6-muscle screen has been recommended for both cervical and lumbosacral radiculopathies.[32] This was based predominantly on prior studies looking at a root screen with or without paraspinal muscles in the cervical and lumbosacral regions. The sensitivity difference among 5-muscle, 6-muscle, and 7-muscle screening algorithms was compared along with various NEE parameters.[36,37] PWs, fibrillations, complex repetitive discharges, high-amplitude, long-duration motor unit action potentials (MUAPs), and reduced recruitment were analyzed. Radiculopathy was considered confirmed when 2 or more muscles from the same root but different peripheral nerves showed any of these findings or when the paraspinal muscles demonstrated fibrillation potentials, PWs, or complex repetitive discharges. The 6-muscle screens were 94% to 99% sensitive in detecting radiculopathy, with the higher range being when paraspinal muscles were included in the screen. Screens can serve as valid initial work-ups, but additional muscles should be examined to confirm the diagnosis.

Paraspinal muscle involvement can be a useful tool to support intraspinal disease and rule out extraspinal causes of motor symptoms, such as plexopathy, but there are limitations of paraspinal muscle NEE examination. Paraspinal abnormalities occur in other disorders, such as motor neuron disease and necrotizing myopathies. Fibrillation potentials or PWs rarely can occur in normal individuals, particularly in the lumbosacral region.[38] The segmental innervation to these muscles can overlap by up to 6 segments in some cases, and thus abnormalities at the C7 vertebral level may not correlate to C7 root pathology.[38,39] Iatrogenic injury during spinal surgery can result in permanent denervation, and fibrillation potentials may persist indefinitely rendering them unreliable when assessing acute or subacute symptoms. In routine clinical practice, paraspinal muscles are not sampled if prior surgery has been performed near the root level of interest.

ACUTE VERSUS CHRONIC RADICULOPATHY

MUAP morphology and the presence or absence of fibrillation potentials help define the age of a radiculopathy. Each of these changes takes time to develop, and the changes seen during NEE need to be correlated with the time of symptom onset. When interpreting the NEE changes, the wording used to describe them also matters and has been a source of debate.[40] In a 2014 study, various terminology was used to describe whether a radiculopathy occurred recently (days to weeks) or in the more distant past (months to years) and if there was evidence of an active or ongoing lesion. Referring providers were asked to interpret this terminology with variable results. Describing the age of a root lesion with words like "acute" to mean days to weeks and "chronic" to mean months to years yielded reliable understanding and is recommended. To indicate whether the lesion still is occurring at the time of NEE, it is recommended to use a qualifier, such as "active" or "inactive." Without these qualifiers, non–EMG-trained physicians had confusion correctly interpreting the EMG report.

In an axonal lesion of less than 3 weeks, insufficient time may have elapsed for the development of abnormal spontaneous activity and MUAP morphology is normal. Occasionally, abnormal insertional activity in the form of very brief trains of PWs may be seen in myotome-specific muscles that could suggest very recent motor axon loss.

After 3 weeks, fibrillation potentials and PWs develop and their presence suggests an active lesion. If the MUAP morphology is normal, this is qualified as an acute, active radiculopathy.

Although axonal lesions produce the most reliable NEE changes, demyelinating lesions also can occur. A demyelinating root lesion with prominent conduction block in the absence of axon loss change (ie, fibrillation potentials) may be suspected when clinical weakness is present; reduced recruitment of normal MUAPs is seen in a muscle whose distal CMAP is normal.

In more chronic root lesions with axonal loss, surviving motor axons attempt to reinnervate denervated muscle fibers via collateral sprouting. This typically occurs between 6 weeks and 26 weeks after the initial root injury. During initial reinnervation, the morphologic appearance of MUAPs is polyphasic and they may be unstable due to immaturity of newly formed neuromuscular junctions. As new neuromuscular junctions stabilize and reinnervation becomes complete, MUAPs take on their final chronic appearance of increased duration and amplitude with a reduced recruitment pattern. When these MUAPs are seen, the lesion is qualified as chronic. Abnormal spontaneous activity seen with chronic MUAPs is indicative of a chronic, active lesion. Alternatively, the absence of abnormal spontaneous activity indicates the lesion is chronic, inactive. Sometimes, very distal muscles never fully reinnervate following root injury. This chronic muscle fiber denervation can result in persistent fibrillation potentials and does not necessarily indicate an active lesion. In these circumstances, it may not be possible to reliably determine if a lesion is active or inactive. If there is further uncertainty, stating that "it is unclear whether there is ongoing nerve root injury" is appropriate.[40]

Single-fiber EMG has been used to study the course of reinnervation of chronic radiculopathy.[41–43] One study evaluated 32 patients with EMG-confirmed chronic radiculopathy based on increased amplitude and duration MUAPs with decreased recruitment. Jitter analysis was performed on the most severely affected muscle, with the most commonly studied muscles in descending order being tibialis anterior, triceps, medial gastrocnemius, vastus lateralis, and rectus femoris. Abnormal mean jitter values were found in 75% of patients with chronic MUAPs on conventional EMG and in 100% of patients where fibrillation potentials were identified. It was concluded, however, that increased jitter was not a reliable measurement and should be avoided in chronic denervated muscles.

CERVICAL RADICULOPATHY

Most muscles have more than 1 root innervation. Although the C5-T1 motor nerve roots are assessed easily on NEE, segmental innervation of a muscle may vary between individuals and important anatomic variations specific to the brachial plexus occur in up to half of all individuals.[44] In those with a prefixed brachial plexus, C4 contributes to traditionally C5-innervated muscles, and, in a postfixed brachial plexus, T2 nerve roots contribute to T1-innervated muscles.

A typical root screen for cervical radiculopathy might include first dorsal interosseous, flexor pollicis longus, extensor indicis proprius, pronator teres, triceps, biceps, and deltoid, effectively covering C5-8. If a radicular distribution of fibrillation potentials is noted during the root screen, the paraspinal muscles also is evaluated. Depending on the root level in question, NCSs and muscles could be added to the root screen study (**Table 3**). In a recent study of 114 patients with an infraspinatus muscle weakness, 16 were found to have C4/5/6 structural (disc herniation or spondylosis) radiculopathy as the cause. They found that in these patients, deltoid was

Table 3
Needle electromyography and nerve conduction abnormalities in cervical radiculopathies

Root	Commonly Affected	Nerve Conduction Study Considerations
C5	Deltoid Biceps Infraspinatus Brachioradialis Rhomboid major	Axillary or musculocutaneous CMAP amplitudes
C6	Deltoid Biceps Infraspinatus Brachioradialis Pronator teres Triceps	A normal amplitude lateral antebrachial cutaneous SNAP reflects an intact C6 DRG, from which it typically is derived.
C7	Triceps > pronator teres Anconeus Flexor carpi radialis Extensor carpi radialis	No reliable studies
C8	First dorsal interosseous Extensor indicis proprius Flexor pollicis longus	Ulnar SNAP is characteristically normal and helps rule out ulnar mononeuropathy and lower trunk/medial cord brachial plexopathy. Medial antebrachial cutaneous SNAP can be obtained to rule out a lower trunk plexopathy and true neurogenic thoracic outlet syndrome.

affected most severely, followed by infraspinatus and then biceps.[45] This underscores the importance of including infraspinatus if a C5/6 radiculopathy is suspected, which increases diagnostic yield because biceps may be normal on NEE in more than 50% of patients.

LUMBOSACRAL RADICULOPATHY

At the lumbosacral root levels, the L5 and S1 root distributions are the most common patterns on NEE. Due to the long length of descent for root fibers in the cauda equina through the central canal for multiple spinal segments, however, the correlation with the spinal level of root damage is not discernible by NEE. For example, a lateral disc herniation at the L2-3 spinal level can produce an L2 or L3 radiculopathy, whereas a central herniation at the same level can produce an L4, L5, or S1 radiculopathy. A study of 14 patients demonstrated that upper lumbar stenosis from L1-L4 resulted most commonly in abnormalities in L5 and S1 myotomes.[46]

A lumbosacral radiculopathy root screen may include tibialis posterior or flexor digitorum longus, medial gastrocnemius, tibialis anterior, rectus femoris or vastus lateralis, and gluteus medius or tensor fascia lata. If peroneal and tibial CMAP amplitudes are reduced, EDB and abductor hallucis may be added to evaluate for distal-proximal gradient of motor axon loss when polyneuropathy is in the differential diagnosis. Additional muscles may be examined when needle abnormalities are found to establish a diagnosis more confidently (**Table 4**). Identification of abnormalities in proximal muscles helps support a diagnosis and exclude mimics such as sciatic and peroneal mononeuropathy. This can be important particularly in elderly patients in whom absent sensory responses might be a normal finding. It is important to recall that a low or absent superficial peroneal SNAP does not reliably exclude an L5

Table 4
Needle electromyography and nerve conduction abnormalities in lumbosacral radiculopathies

Root	Commonly Affected	Nerve Conduction Study Considerations
L2-3	Rectus femoris Vastus medialis Vastus lateralis Iliacus Adductor longus	Saphenous and lateral femoral cutaneous SNAPs can be performed to exclude lumbar plexopathy. Femoral CMAP (rectus femoris) amplitudes may be low.
L4	Rectus Femoris Adductor Longus (tibialis anterior)	Femoral CMAP (rectus femoris) amplitudes may be low.
L5	EDB Tibialis posterior Tibialis anterior Gluteus medius Peroneus longus Extensor hallucis longus Semitendinosus/semimembranosus	Fibular motor (EDB and tibialis anterior) recording
S1	Medial gastrocnemius Short head biceps femoris Gluteus maximus Abductor hallucis	

radiculopathy given the common intraspinal involvement of the L5 DRG.[12] Fibrillation potentials in a myotomal distribution should trigger paraspinal muscle examination.

THORACIC RADICULOPATHY

Thoracic radiculopathy is uncommon.[47] From an EDX standpoint, it is difficult to confirm with a high degree of confidence due to the overlapping multisegment innervation of the paraspinal muscles and rectus abdominus muscles. The NEE approach should include both thoracic paraspinal muscles and relevant levels of the rectus abdominis muscles. The paraspinal examination often is hampered by poor relaxation, precluding reliable assessment of spontaneous activity. Studying the upper, mid, and lower rectus abdominis muscles often is more productive, assessing for both spontaneous activity and MUAP changes.

T1 radiculopathy can be assessed by examination of APB. Flexor pollicis longus also can have significant T1 innervation, but both muscles also can have C8 contributions.[48,49] With T1 radiculopathy, APB shows significant chronic and/or active motor axon loss in the absence of features, suggesting carpal tunnel syndrome. Normal medial antebrachial cutaneous sensory response excludes true neurogenic thoracic outlet syndrome.[50,51]

SUMMARY

EMG is an important tool used to assist in the diagnosis of radiculopathy. NEE is the most sensitive and specific portion of the study in this regard. Finding spontaneous activity and/or MUAP morphologic changes in 2 different muscles of the same myotome, but with different peripheral nerve innervation, supports an EDX of motor radiculopathy. A 6-muscle NEE root screen approach is optimal. Understanding the limitations is important, including the inability to assess sensory-only symptoms. Thus, a normal EMG does not preclude the presence of radiculopathy.

Finally, clear and precise wording of the diagnostic interpretation is required to convey meaning, minimize confusing terminology, and provide proper direction for subsequent patient care.

CLINICS CARE POINTS

- When performing NEE in suspected radiculopathy and neurogenic MUAPs are seen, sample additional muscles innervated by the same root but a different peripheral nerve when possible.
- When radiculopathy is suspected but sensory conduction responses are reduced in amplitude or absent, consider alternative diagnoses.
- Avoid NEE of the paraspinal muscles if posterior spine surgery has been performed in the area of interest.
- A normal EMG study does not exclude radiculopathy as the cause of clinical symptoms, particularly in sensory predominant cases.

DISCLOSURE

The authors have nothing to disclose.

REFERENCES

1. Shea PA, Woods WW, Werden DH. Electromyography in diagnosis of nerve root compression syndrome. Arch Neurol Psychiatry 1950;64:3–104.
2. Zambelis T. The usefulness of electrodiagnostic consultation in an outpatient clinic. J Clin Neurosci 2019;67:59–61.
3. Barrette K, Levin J, Miles D, et al. The value of electrodiagnostic studies in predicting treatment outcomes for patients with spine pathologies. Phys Med Rehabil Clin N Am 2018;29(4):681–7.
4. Haig AJ, Tzeng HM, LeBreck DB. The value of electrodiagnostic consultation for patients with upper extremity nerve complaints: a prospective comparison with the history and physical examination. Arch Phys Med Rehabil 1999;80:1273–81.
5. Hamanishi C, Tanaka S. Dorsal root ganglia in the lumbosacral region observed from the axial views of MRI. Spine 1993;18:1753–6.
6. Kikuchi S, Sato K, Konno S, et al. Anatomic and radiographic study of dorsal root ganglia. Spine 1994;19:6–11.
7. Dumitru D, Zwarts M. Radiculopathies. In: Dumitru D, Amato A, Zwarts M, editors. Electrodiagnostic medicine. Philadelphia: Hanley Belfus Inc; 2002. p. 713–76.
8. Yabuki S, Kikuchi S. Positions of dorsal root ganglia in the cervical spine: an anatomic and clinical study. Spine 1996;21:1513–7.
9. Wilbourn AJ, Aminoff MJ. AAEE Minimonograph #32: The electrophysiologic examination in patients with radiculopathies. Muscle Nerve 1988;11:1099–114.
10. Chen S, Andary M, Buschbacher R, et al. Electrodiagnostic reference values for upper and lower limb nerve conduction studies in adult populations. Muscle Nerve 2016;54(3):371–7.
11. Dillingham T, Chen S, Andary M, et al. Establishing high quality reference values for nerve conduction studies: a report from the normative data task force of the American Association of Neuromuscular & Electrodiagnostic Medicine. Muscle Nerve 2016;54(3):366–70.

12. Levin KH. L5 radiculopathy with reduced superficial peroneal sensory responses: intraspinal and extraspinal causes. Muscle Nerve 1998;21:3–7.

13. Mondelli M, Aretini A, Arrigucci U, et al. Sensory nerve action potential amplitude is rarely reduced in lumbosacral radiculopathy due to herniated disc. Clin Neurophysiol 2013;124(2):405–9.

14. Benecke R, Conrad B. The Distal Sensory Nerve Action Potential as a Diagnostic Tool for the Differentiation of Lesions in Dorsal Roots and Peripheral Nerves. J Neurol 1980;223:231–9.

15. Tavee JO, Polston D, Zhou L, et al. Sural sensory nerve action potential, epidermal nerve fiber density, and quantitative sudomotor axon reflex in healthy elderly. Muscle Nerve 2014;49(4):564–9.

16. Levin KH, Stevens JC, Daube JR. Superficial peroneal nerve conduction studies for electromyographic diagnosis. Muscle Nerve 1986;9(4):322–6.

17. Li JM, Tavee J. Electrodiagnosis of radiculopathy. Handbook Clin Neurol 2019; 161(3):305–16.

18. Berger AR, Sharma K, Lipton RB. Comparison of motor conduction abnormalities in lumbosacral radiculopathy and axonal polyneuropathy. Muscle Nerve 1999;22: 1053–7.

19. McNeish B, Hearn S, Craig A, et al. Motor amplitudes may predict electromyography-confirmed radiculopathy in patients referred for radiating limb pain. Muscle Nerve 2019;59(5):561–6.

20. Kim HJ, Nemani VM, Piyaskulkaew C, et al. Cervical radiculopathy: incidence and treatment of 1,420 consecutive cases. Asian Spine J 2016;10:231–7.

21. Polston DW. Cervical Radiculopathy. Neurol Clin 2007;25:373–85.

22. Daube JR, Rubin DI. AANEM Monograph: Needle Electromyography. Muscle Nerve 2009;39:244–70.

23. Zheng C, Liang J, Nie C, et al. F-waves of peroneal and tibial nerves in the differential diagnosis and follow-up evaluation of L5 and S1 radiculopathies. Eur Spine J 2018;27(8):1734–43.

24. Gill NW 3rd, Ruediger TM, Gochis RD, et al. Test-retest reliability of the ulnar F-wave minimum latency in normal adults. Electromyogr Clin Neurophysiol 1999;39(4):195–200.

25. Pinheiro DS, Manzano GM, Nobrega JA. Reproducibility in nerve conduction studies and F-wave analysis. Clin Neurophysiol 2008;119(9):2070–3.

26. Cho SC, Ferrante MA, Levin KH, et al. Utility of electrodiagnostic testing in evaluating patients with lumbosacral radiculopathy: an evidence-based review. Muscle Nerve 2010;42:276–82.

27. Taga A, Poma G, Cattaneo L, et al. Radial Nerve F-wave reference values with surface electrodes from the anconeus muscle. Muscle Nerve 2019;59(2):244–6.

28. Papathanasiou ES, Zamba E, Papacostas SS. Radial nerve F-waves: normative values with surface recording from the extensor indicis muscle. Clin Neurophysiol 2001;112(1):145–52.

29. Tsao B, Levin KH. Comparison of surgical and electrodiagnostic findings in single root lumbosacral radiculopathies. Muscle Nerve 2003;27:60–4.

30. Emad MR, Momeninejad H, Tahvildari BP, et al. A comparison of H-reflex in the triceps surae muscle group in patients with S1 radiculopathy. Somatosens Mot Res 2017;34(4):213–8.

31. Jankus WR, Robinson LR, Little JW. Normal limits of side-to-side H-reflex amplitude variability. Arch Phys Med Rehabil 1994;75:3–6.

32. Dillingham TR, Annaswamy TM, Plastaras CT. AANEM monograph: Evaluation of persons with suspected lumbosacral and cervical radiculopathy:

Electrodiagnostic assessment and implications for treatment and outcomes (Part 1). Muscle Nerve 2020;62(4):462–73.

33. Tong HC, Haig AJ, Yamakawa KS, et al. Specificity of needle electromyography for lumbar radiculopathy and plexopathy in 55 to79 year old asymptomatic subjects. Am J Phys Med Rehabil 2006;85(11):908–12.

34. Tong HC. Specificity of needle electromyography for lumbar radiculopathy in 55 to 79 year old subjects with low back pain and sciatica without stenosis. Am J Phys Med Rehabil 2011;90(3):233–8.

35. American Association of Electrodiagnostic Medicine. Guidelines in electrodiagnostic medicine. The scope of electrodiagnostic medicine. Muscle Nerve Suppl 1999;8:S5–12.

36. Dillingham TR, Lauder TD, Andary M, et al. Identification of cervical radiculopathies: optimizing the electromyographic screen. Am J Physmed Rehabil 2001;80:84–91.

37. Dillingham TR, Lauder TD, Andary M, et al. Identifying lumbosacral radiculopathies: an optimal electromyographic screen. Am J Phys Med Rehabil 2000;79:496–503.

38. Dumitru D, Diaz CA, King JC. Prevalence of denervation in paraspinal and foot intrinsic musculature. Am J Phys Med Rehabil 2001;80(7):482–90.

39. Gough J, Koepke G. Electromyographic determination of motor root levels in erector spinae muscles. Arch Phys Med Rehabil 1966;47:9–11.

40. Mauricio EA, Dimberg EL, Kennelly KD, et al. Improving referring physicians' understanding of electromyography reports when qualifying radiculopathies: A need for standardized terminology. Muscle Nerve 2014;49(1):129–30.

41. Kouyoumdjian JA, Ronchi LG, de Faria FO. Jitter evaluation in denervation and reinnervation in 32 cases of chronic radiculopathy. Clin Neurophysiol Pract 2020;5:165–72.

42. Pond A, Marcante A, Zanato R, et al. History, mechanisms and clinical value of fibrillation analyses in muscle denervation and reinnervation by single fiber electromyography and dynamic echomyography. Eur J Transl Myol 2014;24(1):3297.

43. Wiechers D. Single fiber EMG evaluation in denervation and reinnervation. Muscle Nerve 1990;13(9):829–32.

44. Uysal II, Seker M, Karabulut AK, et al. Brachial plexus variations in human fetuses. Neurosurgery 2003;53:676–84.

45. Seror P, Roren A, Lefevre-Colau MM. Infraspinatus muscle palsy involving suprascapular nerve, brachial plexus or cervical roots related to inflammatory or mechanical issues: Experience of 114 cases. Clin Neurophysiol 2020;50:103–11.

46. Park JH, Chung SG, Kim K. Electrodiagnostic characteristics of upper lumbar stenosis: Discrepancy between neurological and structural levels. Muscle Nerve 2020;61(5):580–6.

47. Longstreth GF. Diabetic thoracic polyradiculopathy. Best Pract Res Clin Gastroenterol 2005;19(2):275–81.

48. Levin K. Neurological manifestations of compressive radiculopathy of the first thoracic root. Neurology 1999;53(5):1149–51.

49. Radecki J, Feinberg JH, Zimmer ZR. T1 Radiculopathy: Electrodiagnostic evaluation. HSS J 2009;5:73–7.

50. Ferrante MA, Ferrante ND. AANEM Monograph: The thoracic outlet syndromes: Part 1. Overview of the thoracic outlet syndromes and review of true neurogenic thoracic outlet syndrome. Muscle Nerve 2017;55:782–93.

51. Maggiano H, Levin KH, Wilbourn AJ. Relationship between medial antebrachial cutaneous sensory and median motor responses in brachial plexopathy. Muscle Nerve 1993;16:113–4.

Electrodiagnostic Assessment of Plexopathies

Priya Sai Dhawan, MD, FRCPC[1]

KEYWORDS

- Brachial plexopathy • Lumbosacral plexopathy • Electrodiagnostic studies
- Electromyography • Nerve conduction studies

KEY POINTS

- Injury to the brachial and lumbosacral plexus may result from trauma, external compression by surrounding structures, inflammatory or hereditary peripheral nerve disorders, infiltration by malignancy, or delayed damage from radiation therapy.
- Pain, weakness, and atrophy are commonly encountered in patients with brachial and lumbosacral plexopathy.
- Knowledge of plexus anatomy and a systematic electrodiagnostic approach allows for precise and efficient localization and may help determine the underlying cause.
- Assessment of sensory nerve action potentials and needle examination of paraspinal muscles are valuable differentiating disorders of nerve roots from plexopathies.
- Co-existing nerve root avulsion, presence of low-amplitude compound motor action potentials, evidence of significant denervation on needle examination, and inability to voluntarily recruit motor units 4 to 6 months after a traumatic plexopathy are poor prognosticating factors for spontaneous recovery.

INTRODUCTION

Disorders of the brachial and lumbosacral plexus present as a challenge for the clinician and electromyographer. These conditions are rare, may present with nonspecific clinical features, involve intricate anatomy, and may mimic more commonly encountered nerve root or peripheral nerve disorders. The clinician must be vigilant about the possibility of a plexopathy; to do so requires an understanding of structural plexus anatomy, innervation patterns, and associated pathologic entities. A stepwise electrodiagnostic (EDX) approach allows for efficient localization and can provide important information about severity, prognosis, and, on occasion cause. This article reviews EDX features that help to identify plexopathies, guides the electromyographer toward a systematic evaluation and highlights EDX features unique to specific disorders of the plexus.

Department of Neurology, University of British Columbia, Koerner Pavilion, UBC Hospital, S192-2211 Westbrook Mall, North Vancouver, British Columbia V6T 2B5, Canada
[1] Present address: 340-138 E 13th Street, North Vancouver, BC V7L 0E5, Canada.
E-mail address: priya.dhawan@vch.ca

Neurol Clin 39 (2021) 997–1014
https://doi.org/10.1016/j.ncl.2021.06.006
0733-8619/21/Crown Copyright © 2021 Published by Elsevier Inc. All rights reserved.

HISTORY AND PHYSICAL EXAMINATION

A thorough clinical history and examination are necessary first steps in the assessment of a patient with extremity weakness and sensory loss; EDX confirmation of a plexopathy will more likely be accomplished if suspected clinically. Plexopathies are frequently accompanied by exquisite neuropathic pain, particularly when caused by inflammatory or neoplastic processes.[1] Although sensory symptoms may follow dermatomal patterns, they are often poorly localizable.[2] Weakness and atrophy are typically present, reflecting the axonal nature of most plexopathies. Subacute and self-limiting pain and weakness may suggest an inflammatory cause, a progressive course implicates a possible malignancy or other structural process,[3] and acute onset of stuttering symptoms may raise suspicion for ischemia.[4]

Important historical features include recent trauma, antecedent illness, history of malignancy, comorbid connective tissue diseases, prior radiation therapy, constitutional symptoms such as weight loss, and a history of diabetes. For example, a diabetic patient who presents with anterior thigh pain, hip flexor and quadriceps weakness, thoracic pain with abdominal wall weakness, and rapid, profound weight loss is likely to have a diabetic thoracic and lumbosacral radiculoplexus neuropathy.[5] Other examination findings may suggest potential causes; for example, Horner syndrome and a palpable axillary mass implicates involvement of T1 fibers and would raise the possibility of a Pancoast tumor.

ELECTRODIAGNOSTIC APPROACH TO PLEXOPATHIES

EDX studies are an important step in the confirmation of a clinically suspected plexopathy. Goals of the EDX evaluation are to (1) confirm localization to the plexus, (2) exclude nerve root or peripheral nerve pathology, (3) precisely localize to the site within the plexus, (4) identify subclinical involvement of other plexus regions, (5) characterize the pathophysiology as axonal or demyelinating, (6) define severity, (7) guide prognosis, and (8) potentially shed light on a cause.

A high clinical suspicion of a plexopathy before beginning EDX studies is important to guide the evaluation. Routinely performed nerve conduction studies (NCS), such as the median and ulnar sensory NCS, primarily evaluate the lateral and medial cords but not the posterior cord.[6] Therefore, less commonly performed NCS (eg, musculocutaneous, medial and lateral antebrachial cutaneous, superficial radial, or saphenous in the leg) are often required for a complete assessment of the brachial or lumbosacral plexus.[2] At minimum, NCS in the distribution of clinical weakness or sensory loss, and needle examination of clinically weak muscles should be performed. Using a systematic approach to NCS and needle examination allows for a more complete and reliable assessment of abnormalities within the plexus.

Sensory Nerve Action Potentials

The findings on sensory nerve action potentials (SNAPs) are particularly important in the EDX confirmation of a plexopathy and exclusion of root pathology. Because most nerve root injuries are preganglionic, they result in preservation of distal SNAPs; by contrast, the plexi are formed by fibers distal to the dorsal root ganglion, and Wallerian degeneration of the sensory axons results in low SNAPs.[2] Therefore, the presence of abnormal SNAPs helps to distinguish a plexopathy from a radiculopathy, particularly in the upper extremity.[7] Side-to-side SNAP comparison is important, particularly in a younger patient with borderline SNAP amplitudes or in sensory NCS for which normal values do not exist. Typically, a 50% amplitude difference between sides is considered abnormal.

Motor Nerve Conduction Studies

Compound muscle action potentials (CMAPs) are often low amplitude in plexopathies associated with axonal damage. There may also be mild (non-demyelinating range) slowing of conduction velocity, prolongation of distal latency, and prolongation of F-waves.[6] Because low CMAPs can also be seen in radiculopathies or mononeuropathies, they do not help to distinguish a plexopathy from other localizations. Rarely, a conduction block or temporal dispersion may be present across the plexus, indicating areas of focal demyelination (ie, radiation plexopathy or focal compression).[8] Caution should be used in interpreting the presence or absence of a proximal block at the axilla or Erb point because submaximal stimulation may mimic conduction block, and costimulation of adjacent nerves may interfere with isolated CMAP recording (ie, stimulation of the median nerve at Erb point may produce a mixed ulnar and median CMAP when recording over the thenar eminence).[6]

Needle Examination

A thorough, organized needle examination with examination of muscles from each individual trunk, cord, and peripheral nerve is important to help localize the site of involvement.[2] A common approach is to initially examine muscles from each nerve root and major peripheral nerve and further target the study based on abnormalities. Abnormalities in certain proximal limb innervated by nerves derived directly from the roots (eg, rhomboids and serratus anterior) and paraspinal muscles help to differentiate a radiculopathy from a plexopathy.

The findings on needle examination reflect the severity and chronicity of injury, as well as the degree of recovery from reinnervation. Fibrillation potentials are common, given the typical pathophysiology of axonal loss, and reduced recruitment of long duration motor unit potentials (MUPs) indicates reinnervation. Some discharges have diagnostic significance; for example, myokymic discharges are associated with radiation plexopathy,[9] or "nascent" MUPs signify very early reinnervation in severe traumatic plexopathies.[10]

BRACHIAL PLEXOPATHIES

The brachial plexus is a complex network of nerves extending from the lower neck, across the shoulder and toward the axilla (**Fig. 1**). Disorders causing brachial plexopathies include inflammatory conditions, infiltration by malignancy, direct trauma, external compression from surrounding structures, and hereditary conditions (**Table 1**).[1,3–5,11–24] The brachial plexus is susceptible to external injury due to its length and, in some locations, superficial location. Shorter, less protected cervical nerve roots are more vulnerable to traction than the plexus and may become avulsed in traumatic upper extremity injuries. The trunks lie superficially before they divide into divisions deep to the clavicle and consequently are frequently exposed to external trauma. Trunk injuries are more common than cord injuries and typically confer a worse prognosis. Pathology involving adjacent neck, axillary, or mediastinal structures (bones such as the humerus and clavicle, blood vessels, apex of the lung, lymph nodes) may externally compress or infiltrate the closely situated plexus.[2]

The anatomy has been well described[6]; however, a few salient points are highlighted, as they relate to EDX studies:

- The plexus is derived of fibers from the ventral rami of C5-T1 nerve roots, although a small percentage of the population has derivation from C4 (prefixed) or T2 (postfixed) roots.

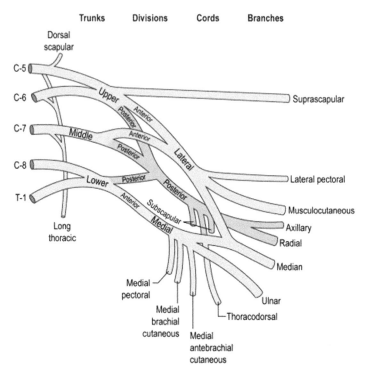

Fig. 1. Brachial plexus anatomy. (*From* Preston D, Shapiro B. Electromyography and Neuromuscular Disorders: Clinical-Electrophysiologic Correlations, Edition 2. Philadelphia: Elsevier Butterworth-Heinemann; 2005; with permission.)

- The dorsal rami of cervical nerve roots (innervating the cervical paraspinal muscles) and nerves emerging directly from cervical roots (dorsal scapular nerve [rhomboid complex and levator scapulae], the long thoracic nerve [serratus anterior], the phrenic nerve [diaphragm], and the nerve to the subclavian muscle [C5-6]) are not part of the plexus.[21]
- The roots join to form *trunks*, *divisions*, and *cords* before terminating as individual peripheral nerves. Rarely do disorders involve the divisions in isolation; thus localization is usually focused on the trunks or cords.
- The main terminal peripheral nerves in the upper extremity are formed from the plexus. **Table 2** details the innervation of major upper extremity muscles by nerve root, trunk, cord, and peripheral nerve.

Different motor and sensory NCS can be used to test specific segments of the brachial plexus and, when performed in a technically reliable manner, help to accurately reflect plexus localization and pathology.[12] An approach to the EDX evaluation of the brachial plexus is outlined in **Table 3**.

ELECTRODIAGNOSTIC FEATURES IN SPECIFIC BRACHIAL PLEXOPATHIES
Traumatic Brachial Plexopathy

Trauma to the brachial plexus may occur as a result of injury in the birth canal,[19] penetrating trauma, falls, and high-velocity injuries such as motor vehicle accidents.[25] Recently, upper trunk brachial plexopathy has been described as a consequence of

Table 1
Disorders affecting the brachial or lumbosacral plexus

	Brachial	Lumbosacral
Inflammatory	Post-surgical inflammatory radiculoplexus neuropathy	Post-surgical inflammatory radiculoplexus neuropathy Diabetic/non-diabetic lumbosacral radiculoplexus neuropathy
	Idiopathic inflammatory brachial plexopathy (eg, Parsonage-Turner syndrome)	
	Paraneoplastic	Paraneoplastic
	Focal or multifocal chronic inflammatory demyelinating polyradiculoneuropathy (CIDP)	CIDP
	Neurosarcoidosis	Neurosarcoidosis
Neoplastic	Metastatic infiltration (eg, breast, lung, sarcoma)	Metastatic infiltration (eg, prostate, cervix, colorectal, bladder, sarcoma)
	Neurolymphomatosis	Neurolymphomatosis
	Pancoast tumor, axillary mass	Inguinal mass
	Peripheral nerve tumors (eg, schwannoma, perineurioma, neurofibroma, malignant nerve sheath tumor)	Peripheral nerve tumors (eg, schwannoma, perineurioma, neurofibroma, malignant nerve sheath tumor)
Hereditary	Hereditary intermittent brachial plexopathy Hereditary neuropathy with liability to pressure palsies from PMP22 deletion (ie,: "backpack palsy")	
Trauma	Birth injury (eg, Erb, Klumpke)	Hip and sacroiliac fracture or dislocation
	High-velocity blunt or penetrating injury (ie,: motor vehicle accident, stretch injury)	Pregnancy and parturition
	Shoulder fracture or dislocation	
Structural	Neurogenic thoracic outlet syndrome	Retroperitoneal hematoma/abscess
	Poststernotomy	
	Radiation	Radiation "Insulin neuritis," a self-limiting plexopathy associated with rapid glycemic correction in new diabetics
Vascular	Ischemia (eg, arterial thromboembolism, peripheral vascular disease)	Ischemia (eg, arterial thromboembolism, peripheral vascular disease)
	Primary or systemic peripheral nerve vasculitis	Primary or systemic peripheral nerve vasculitis
	Subclavian aneurysm	Abdominal aneurysm

Table 2
Muscles innervated by brachial plexus segments (trunk, cord, peripheral nerve)

	Upper Trunk (C5-C6)	Middle Trunk (C6-C7-C8)	Lower Trunk (C8-T1)
	Suprascapular Infraspinatus Supraspinatus		
Lateral Cord	Musculocutaneous Biceps Brachialis Lateral pectoral Pectoralis major	Median (C6-7) Pronator teres Flexor carpi radialis	
Posterior Cord	Axillary Deltoid Teres major Radial (C6) Brachioradialis Supinator Triceps Subscapular nerves Subscapularis	Radial (C7) Triceps Extensor carpi radialis Anconeus Extensor digitorum communis Extensor carpi ulnaris Thoracodorsal Latissimus dorsi	Radial (C8) Extensor indicis proprius Extensor carpi ulnaris
Medial Cord			Ulnar (C8) First dorsal interosseous Abductor digiti minimi Flexor carpi ulnaris Flexor digitorum profundus Median (T1) Abductor pollicis brevis Flexor pollicis longus Medial pectoral Pectoralis minor Pectoralis major

Adapted from Rubin DI. Brachial and lumbosacral plexopathies: A review. Clin Neurophysiol Pract. 2020;5:173–193. Published 2020 Aug 13. https://doi.org/10.1016/j.cnp.2020.07.005; with permission.

the prone positioning required in the management of patients with SARS-CoV-2.[26] The mechanism of injury may inform localization; lateral movements of the head away from the shoulder may result in upper trunk injury, whereas overhead abduction of the arm predominately affects the lower trunk.[25] The supraclavicular structures (trunks) are vulnerable to traumatic stretch injury. In some patients, an underlying diffuse peripheral nervous system disorder may predispose the patient to additional compression plexopathies. For example, EDX studies in persons developing upper trunk plexopathies after heavy backpack use (ie, "rucksack palsy") may show subclinical features that suggest hereditary neuropathy with liability to pressure palsies, such as

Table 3
Suggested electrodiagnostic approach for brachial plexopathies

	Studies	Notes

Sensory NCS	Median (antidromic)
	Ulnar (antidromic)
	Superficial radial
	Lateral antebrachial
	  cutaneous (for
	  suspected upper trunk)
	Median antebrachial
	  cutaneous (for
	  suspected lower trunk)
		• Study each nerve with
		  weakness or sensory loss
		• Perform side-to-side
		  comparison in young
		  patients with low normal
		  or borderline responses
		• Stimulation of ulnar and
		  median nerves (motor) at
		  the axilla and Erb point

Motor NCS	Median (APB)
	Ulnar (ADM)
	Radial (EDC)
	Median/ulnar
	  F-waves if needed
		can be considered in suspected
		lower trunk or medial cord
		lesions when distal CMAPs
		are normal. A 40% conduction
		block between proximal and
		distal sites is required, given
		technical difficulty of this study.
		Aim for precise stimulator
		placement (watch the muscle
		twitch) and avoid both
		submaximal and overstimulation.
		• Stimulation of
		  musculocutaneous,
		  axillary, suprascapular nerves
		  (motor) can be considered to
		  further support an upper trunk
		  plexopathy

Needle EMG	**Screening**
	Deltoid (upper trunk,
	  posterior cord,
	  axillary, C5-6)
	Biceps (upper trunk,
	  lateral cord,
	  musculocutaneous,
	  C5-6)
	Triceps (upper/middle
	  trunk, posterior cord,
	  radial, C7)
	Pronator teres (middle trunk,
	  lateral cord, median, C6-7)
	First dorsal interosseous
	  (lower trunk,
	  medial cord, ulnar, C8-T1)
	Cervical paraspinals (2 levels)
	Additional
	Brachioradialis
	  (upper trunk,
	  posterior cord,
	  radial, C5-6)
	Extensor digitorum
	  communis (middle trunk,
	  posterior cord, radial C6-8)
		• Study clinically weak muscles
		• Confirmation of a plexopathy
		  requires abnormalities in at
		  least 2 muscles innervated by
		  different nerves
		• When denervation is appreciated,
		  sample other muscles innervated
		  by the same nerve, different root
		  (excludes radiculopathy), as well
		  as muscles by the same root,
		  different nerve (excludes
		  mononeuropathy)
		• If there are abnormalities
		  in a specific trunk or root
		  based on the screening needle
		  examination, test additional
		  muscles innervated by that
		  nerve root to determine whether
		  abnormalities correspond to a
		  specific cord
		• Normal evaluation of rhomboid,
		  serratus anterior, cervical
		  paraspinals, and (if needed)
		  diaphragm allows for exclusion
		  of nerve root pathology

(continued on next page)

Table 3 (continued)	
Studies	**Notes**
Extensor indicis proprius (lower trunk, posterior cord, radial, C8-T1) Flexor pollicis longus (lower trunk, medial cord, median, C8-T1) Rhomboid (C4) Serratus anterior (C5-6-7) Diaphragm (C3-4-5)	• Needle examination of the contralateral side may reveal subclinical disease (typical of inflammatory conditions)

Abbreviations: ABP, abductor pollicis brevis; ADM, adductor digiti minimi; EDC, extensor digitorum communis.

conduction block at sites of compression, slowing of conduction velocity, or subtle distal latency prolongation, prompting genetic analysis of the *PMP22* gene.[18]

Baseline EDX studies should be obtained 3 to 4 weeks following the initial injury, with serial examinations over time to assess for degree of recovery. Reduced recruitment of motor units potentials is often the earliest electrophysiologic abnormality and may be identified almost immediately after acute injury to the brachial plexus. By approximately 7 to 10 days, CMAP and SNAP amplitudes will reach their nadir. Amplitude reductions are comparable to the degree of axonal loss; a robust CMAP in a clinically weak myotome at 7 days favors a neuropraxic injury. Fibrillation potentials are apparent at 3 to 4 weeks after injury followed by large, morphologically complex motor units (signs of reinnervation) after weeks to months.[27]

In pure brachial plexus lesions, rhomboid and serratus anterior should be spared, as should cervical paraspinal muscles.[21] Abnormalities in these muscles suggest additional cervical nerve root avulsion, a consequence of violent traction to the brachial plexus, and typically a poor prognostic factor.[2] Identification of dense fibrillation potentials, low amplitude or absent CMAPs, or inability to activate MUPs 4 to 6 months after injury in a traumatic plexopathy may suggest lack of axonal continuity, conferring poor prognosis[10] and potentially supporting surgical intervention, such as neural decompression, nerve grafting, or tendon transfers.[28] Pan-plexopathies confer a worse prognosis and have variable responses to reconstruction.[25] Evidence of reinnervation in a clinically improving patient may support observation over surgical interventions.[10]

Intraoperative monitoring of nerve action potentials (NAPs) may predict reinnervation earlier than conventional NCS, as the presence of an NAP across a lesion suggests favorable recovery of the nerve with neurolysis as opposed to more aggressive surgical treatments.[25]

Inflammatory Brachial Plexopathy

Inflammatory brachial plexopathies may be idiopathic, para-infectious, post-surgical, or hereditary and present as intense, often self-limiting, pain followed by weakness and atrophy.[29] Involvement of structures outside of the plexus, such as cervical roots or individual nerves, is common.[20] Bilateral, typically asymmetric, involvement may occur in up to 29% of patients[30] and may be subclinical. Neuralgic amyotrophy or "Parsonage-Turner syndrome" may involve the plexus diffusely but there is often patchy, preferential involvement of upper trunk pure motor nerves (axillary and suprascapular), long thoracic, and anterior interosseous nerve fibers.[20] Unilateral or bilateral phrenic nerves may also be affected. Needle examination requires testing many muscles, including less commonly examined muscles such as the flexor pollicis longus or serratus anterior. The presence of dysmorphic features and strong family history may raise suspicion of an autosomal dominant hereditary neuralgic amyotrophy from mutations in the *SPT9* gene, which is clinically and electrodiagnostically indistinguishable from the acquired form.[18]

Neurogenic Thoracic Outlet Syndrome

In neurogenic thoracic outlet syndrome (TOS), the lower trunk of the brachial plexus is compressed by a fibrous band or cervical rib, resulting in sensory loss in the medial hand as well as forearm, weakness of intrinsic hand muscles and occasionally a Horner syndrome; this preferentially involves T1 over C8 fibers, and because thenar muscles receive greater innervation from T1 than C8, the median CMAP is often more affected than the ulnar CMAP.[31] The median sensory responses will be normal, as these sensory fibers pass through upper and middle trunks.[12] The medial antebrachial cutaneous SNAPs are sensitive studies for lower trunk or medial cord plexopathies and may be affected earlier or more severely than more routine ulnar sensory studies.[32]

Neoplastic Brachial Plexopathy

Painful brachial plexopathies from neoplastic disease may occur due to external compression, such as with Pancoast tumor or axillary lymph node enlargement, or direct neural invasion from metastatic disease (eg, neurolymphomatosis, spread from leptomeningeal disease). Peripheral nerve sheath tumors rarely involve the brachial plexus and are typically painless.[14]

Understanding the relationship of the plexus to adjacent structures may allow the electromyographer to predict where pathology may lie. For example, the supraclavicular location of the brachial plexus trunks (particularly the upper trunk) makes these segments vulnerable to inferior growth from a head and neck malignancies, whereas malignant pulmonary neoplasms ("Pancoast tumor") will extend superiorly and invade the lower trunk. Masses in the axilla, from breast cancer or malignant lymphadenopathy, may spare the plexus but affect multiple peripheral nerves at their origin (median, ulnar, radial) and mimic a plexopathy. A paravertebral (ie, chordoma) or epidural tumor near the T1 vertebrae may affect the sympathetic chain and consequently cause a Horner syndrome.[21]

Because of the proximity to mediastinal structures, the lower trunk is most commonly affected and may have similar EDX and clinical features as neurogenic TOS. Medial antebrachial cutaneous responses may be the most sensitive NCS at detecting early or mild involvement of the lower trunk in neoplastic plexopathies. The EDX abnormalities predominately reflect axonal pathology; however, rare cases of proximal conduction block mimicking a focal chronic inflammatory demyelinating polyradiculoneuropathy have been described.[33] Diagnostic imaging (MRI and PET with fludeoxyglucose F 18) is often required to distinguish cases of recurrent neoplasm from radiation plexopathy.[24]

Radiation Plexopathy

Radiation injury to the brachial plexus is an increasingly recognized complication of high-dose (>5000–6000 cGy) radiation to chest wall, axilla, breast, or head and neck structures,[22] with the affected region corresponding with the area of greatest radiation exposure. Fibrotic and microangiopathic ischemic mechanisms have been implicated. Clinical features may occur as early as 1 month after radiation exposure but are more frequently delayed for 1 to 5 years, and may be as long as decades, after exposure. The absence of severe pain may help to distinguish radiation injury from direct neural invasion, but the distribution of weakness does not aid in this distinction.[22] Although some patients may exhibit a degree of improvement or stabilization, slow progression is typical, and the prognosis for spontaneous recovery is poor.

EDX abnormalities are typically unilateral.[34] Although features of axonal loss (low SNAP and CMAP amplitudes, neurogenic motor unit potentials, and scattered fibrillation potentials) predominate on EDX studies, proximal conduction block at Erb point has been reported and is more commonly seen with radiation injury than neoplastic disease.[22] A characteristic needle electromyography feature is the presence of myokymic discharges, which occur in up to 63% of patients.[22]

Similar clinical and EDX features can also occur in radiation-induced lumbosacral plexopathies from abdominal and pelvic radiation. In these cases, injury to the lumbosacral plexus is often bilateral and can involve the upper lumbar or lumbosacral plexus, depending on the site of radiation.

Illustrative Case

A 49-year-old woman was referred for a 3-month history of painful, progressive right upper extremity weakness and sensory loss. Her clinical examination was limited to due pain but her biceps reflex was reduced and there was a palpable mass in the supraclavicular area.

Routine NCS demonstrated an absent superficial radial SNAP and a borderline median SNAP amplitude (15 uV), with a normal ulnar SNAP and median and ulnar motor responses. The contralateral median SNAP amplitude was 32 uV, confirming an abnormality on the symptomatic limb, and the lateral antebrachial cutaneous SNAP amplitude was low on the symptomatic limb (2 uV vs 18 uV). These NCS suggested an upper trunk ± middle trunk brachial plexopathy (**Table 4**). In suspected upper trunk plexopathies, axillary and musculocutaneous CMAPs can also be assessed, but the needle examination is often sufficient for further localization. The needle examination recorded large, polyphasic, occasionally varying MUPs with reduced recruitment and dense fibrillation potentials in the deltoid, biceps, and brachioradialis, with normal findings in the triceps, pronator teres, extensor digitorum, first dorsal interosseous, rhomboid major, and cervical paraspinals. These findings, in combination with abnormal SNAPs, confirmed an upper trunk brachial plexopathy.

MRI of the brachial plexus showed a supraclavicular mass that externally compressed and locally infiltrated the upper trunk of the brachial plexus. Biopsy of the mass confirmed the presence of a B-cell lymphoma, and the patient responded to Rituximab with marked improvements in pain, strength, and sensation.

LUMBOSACRAL PLEXUS

The lumbosacral plexus is a complex network of nerves that is formed by ventral rami of T12-S4 nerve roots (**Fig. 2**). The anatomy has been well described[6]; however, several points are important to consider:

- The lumbosacral plexus is divided into the upper lumbar plexus (T12-L4) and lower lumbosacral plexus (L5-S4), with multiple nerves arising directly off the plexus.
- The upper lumbar plexus lies in the retroperitoneal space and divides within the psoas muscle.[35] Consequently, retroperitoneal pathology (eg, hematoma or

Table 4
NCS corresponding to brachial plexus segments

	Upper Trunk (C5-C6)	Middle Trunk (C6-C7-C8)	Lower Trunk (C8-T1)

Lateral cord	Sensory
	  Median antidromic
	  (thumb, index)
	  Lateral antebrachial
	  cutaneous (forearm)
	Motor
	  Musculocutaneous
	  (biceps)
		Sensory
		  Median
		  antidromic
		  (index, middle)	

Posterior Cord	Sensory
	  Superficial radial
	  (dorsal hand)
	Motor
	  Axillary (deltoid)
		Sensory
		  Superficial
		  radial (
		  dorsal hand)
		Motor
		  Radial (EDC)	

Medial Cord			Sensory
			  Ulnar antidromic
			  (fifth)
			  Dorsal ulnar
			  cutaneous
			  (dorsal hand)
			  Medial antebrachial
			  cutaneous (forearm)
			Motor
			  Median (ABP)
			  Ulnar (ADM, FDI)

Abbreviations: ABP, abductor pollicis brevis; ADM, adductor digiti minimi; EDC, extensor digitorum communis; FDI, first dorsal interosseous.

Adapted from Rubin DI. Brachial and lumbosacral plexopathies: A review. Clin Neurophysiol Pract. 2020;5:173-193. Published 2020 Aug 13. https://doi.org/10.1016/j.cnp.2020.07.005; with permission.

abscess) should be considered in patients presenting with an upper lumbar plexopathy.[36]

- Because the lumbosacral plexus lies deep within the pelvis, it is less vulnerable to penetrating and stretch injuries than the brachial plexus but may still be injured by hip dislocation and anteriorly displaced sacral fracture or dislocation.[37]

Differentiating disorders involving the lumbosacral nerve roots from those involving the plexus is important, as the diagnostic implications of a radiculopathy differ from plexopathy. In some conditions involving the lumbosacral plexus, the pathology extends to involve the roots and peripheral nerves (ie, *radiculoplexus neuropathy*).[3]

GENERAL ELECTROPHYSIOLOGIC FEATURES IN LUMBOSACRAL PLEXOPATHIES

Similar to brachial plexopathies, EDX confirmation of a lumbosacral plexopathy relies on the presence of abnormal SNAPs and a normal needle examination of paraspinal muscles to support a postganglionic process.[38] Sensory studies in the lower extremity may be technically challenging and difficult to interpret, particularly in older individuals in whom SNAPs may be absent normally, and consequently the needle examination is

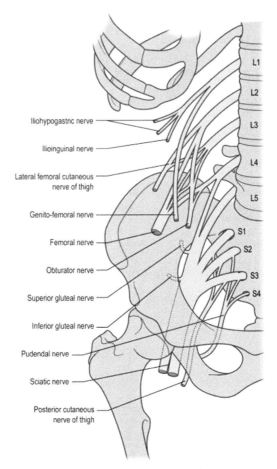

Iliohypogastric nerve

Ilioinguinal nerve

Lateral femoral cutaneous nerve of thigh

Genito-femoral nerve

Femoral nerve

Obturator nerve

Superior gluteal nerve

Inferior gluteal nerve

Pudendal nerve

Sciatic nerve

Posterior cutaneous nerve of thigh

L1 L2 L3 L4 L5 S1 S2 S3 S4

Fig. 2. Lumbosacral plexus anatomy. (*From* Preston D, Shapiro B. Electromyography and Neuromuscular Disorders: Clinical-Electrophysiologic Correlations, Edition 2. Philadelphia: Elsevier Butterworth-Heinemann; 2005; with permission.)

of particular importance (**Table 5**). An approach to the EDX evaluation of the lumbosacral plexus is outlined in **Table 6**. There are several EDX considerations in approach to patients with suspected lumbosacral plexopathies:

- Assessment of upper lumbar plexus with motor NCS is difficult due to the limited number of nerves that can be tested and their deep location within the pelvis. The femoral nerve is the only nerve branching from the lumbar plexus that can be reliably testing with NCS. The deep location of the femoral nerve may require needle stimulation, and care should be taken to avoid the laterally located femoral artery.[3] The saphenous nerve is the terminal sensory branch of the femoral nerve and can be studied with NCS, but they are technically challenging and must be compared with the contralateral side.
- The lateral femoral cutaneous nerve of the thigh courses under the inguinal ligament where it is susceptible to entrapment or compression (*meralgia paresthetica*) and provides sensation to the anterolateral thigh.[35] This nerve does not

Table 5
Lumbosacral plexus segments assessed during nerve conduction studies and needle electromyography

	Nerve	Sensory NCS	Motor NCS	Needle EMG
Upper lumbar plexus	Iliohypogastric *(T12-L1)*	—	—	—
	Ilioinguinal *(L1-L2)*	—	—	—
	Genitofemoral *(L1-2)*	—	—	—
	Femoral *(L2-3-4)*	Saphenous	Femoral	Iliopsoas (partial) Sartorius Pectineus Quadriceps muscles
	Obturator *(L2-3-4)*	—	—	Adductor longus Gracilis Adductor magnus
Lower lumbosacral plexus	Superior gluteal *(L4-5)*	—	—	Gluteus medius
	Inferior gluteal *(L4-S1)*	—	—	Gluteus maximus
	Sciatic *(L4-S2)*	Peroneal Tibial	Sural Medial plantar Lateral plantar	Hamstring muscles Short head of the biceps *(peroneal)* Tibialis anterior *(peroneal)* Medial gastrocnemius *(tibial)* Lateral gastrocnemius *(tibial)* Peroneus longus, tertius *(peroneal)* Posterior tibialis *(tibial)* Soleus Extensor hallucis longus *(peroneal)* Adductor hallucis *(tibial)*
	Pudendal *(S2-3-4)*	—	—	Anal sphincter

branch from the femoral nerve, and therefore involvement of this nerve in conjunction with femoral nerve involvement would be more indicative of a lumbar plexopathy. Although this nerve may be studied by sensory NCS, they are technically challenging, and SNAP amplitudes are normally low and must be compared with the contralateral side.[3]

- Fascicles from the L4 nerve root join L5 to form the lumbosacral trunk, which meets the sacral plexus beyond the pelvic outlet.[35] The location of the trunk makes this vulnerable to trauma from the fetal head during parturition as well as from anteriorly displaced sacral fractures.[11]

Table 6
Suggested electrodiagnostic approach for lumbosacral plexopathies

	Studies	Notes
Sensory NCS	Sural *(S1-2)* Superficial peroneal *(L5)* Saphenous (suspected upper lumbar plexus) *(L3-4)* Lateral femoral cutaneous (suspected upper lumbar plexus) *(L2-3)*	• Study each nerve with weakness or sensory loss • Perform side-to-side comparison in young patients with low normal or borderline responses • The femoral nerve lies deep and may require needle stimulation. • Superficial peroneal and saphenous sensory require side-to-side comparison
Motor NCS	Peroneal (EDB) with F-wave *(L4-5)* Peroneal (TA) *(L4-5)* Tibial (AH) with F-wave *(L5-S2)* Femoral (Vastus) (suspected upper lumbar plexopathy) *(L2-4)*	
Needle EMG	**Screening** Tibialis anterior *(peroneal, L4-5)* Medial gastrocnemius *(tibial, S1/2)* Vastus medialis *(femoral, L3-4)* Tensor fascia latae *(inferior gluteal, L5)* Lumbosacral paraspinals (2 levels) **Additional upper lumbar** Adductor longus *(obturator, L2-3)* Iliopsoas *(L2-4)* Rectus femoris *(L3,4)* **Additional lower lumbosacral** Gluteus medius *(inferior gluteal, L5)* Biceps femoris *(sciatic, L5-S1)* Gluteus maximus *(superior gluteal, S1-2)* Soleus *(tibial, S1-2)* Posterior tibialis *(tibial, L5)* Peroneus longus *(peroneal, L4-5)*	• Study clinically weak muscles • Confirmation of a plexopathy requires abnormalities in at least 2 muscles innervated by different nerves • Needle examination of the contralateral side may reveal subclinical disease (typical of inflammatory conditions) • Needle abnormalities may seem more prominent distally when there is coexisting nerve root, plexus, and peripheral nerve pathology (radiculoplexus neuropathies)

Abbreviations: AH, adductor hallucis; EDB, extensor digitorum brevis; TA, tibialis anterior.

- The sciatic nerve passes deep to the piriformis muscle, a common site of compression, and supplies the hamstring muscles and lateral adductor magnus muscle before bifurcating distally into tibial and peroneal nerves.[35] As some disorders involving the lumbosacral plexus preferentially involve fibers destined for the peroneal nerve, a plexopathy could mimic a peroneal mononeuropathy at the knee. EDX studies are useful in distinguishing the localization; needle examination abnormalities of the short head of the biceps femoris and gluteal muscles localize a process proximal to the peroneal nerve at the knee.[39]

ELECTRODIAGNOSTIC FEATURES IN SPECIFIC LUMBOSACRAL PLEXOPATHIES
Diabetic Lumbosacral Radiculoplexus Neuropathy

Diabetic lumbosacral radiculoplexus neuropathies are typically seen in middle-aged patients with newly diagnosed or relatively well-controlled diabetes. Patients present with rapid and marked weight loss, autonomic impairment, severe neuropathic pain often involving the anterior thigh region and subsequent weakness and atrophy.[5] This immune-mediated microvasculitis is often self-limiting, however may recur on the contralateral side. Treatment with intravenous steroids may reduce the length of pain.[5] Similar pathology has been described in non-diabetic patients and in those with post-surgical inflammatory plexopathy.[16] Rarely, painless variants may exist.

The upper lumbar plexus is most commonly affected, typically with concomitant involvement of lumbar nerve roots (termed *radiculoplexus neuropathy*).[5] The process is patchy, and EDX studies reflect axonal pathology with low CMAP amplitudes and fibrillation potentials. Routinely tested SNAPs may be normal, particularly with upper lumbar plexus pathology, and may mimic a polyradiculopathy.[3] Patients with concomitant thoracic radiculopathy may experience burning thoracic pain with weakness and outpouching of abdominal muscles and demonstrate denervation in thoracic paraspinal muscles.[3]

Illustrative Case

A 69-year-old presented for evaluation of slowly progressive, painless, right leg weakness, and sensory loss over 6 months. He was diagnosed with a right thigh sarcoma 5 years prior, which was treated with resection and radiation. Clinical examination demonstrated weakness in right hip flexors, quadriceps and adductor muscles, patchy sensory loss in the anterior thigh, and an absent right Achilles reflex.

EDX studies demonstrated normal peroneal and tibial CMAP responses and a normal sural SNAP amplitude (12 uV), suggesting integrity of the lower lumbosacral plexus and terminal nerves. Given the robust NCS amplitudes and a weakness pattern suspicious for an upper plexus pathology, additional NCS assessing the lumbar plexus were performed. The femoral CMAP was low (1.4 mV) compared with the unaffected limb (7.2 mV), and the saphenous SNAP was absent (12 uV on the contralateral limb). These NCS findings indicated either an upper lumbar plexopathy or a femoral neuropathy. Needle examination demonstrated fibrillation potentials and reduced recruitment with long duration motor unit potentials in the vastus medialis, adductor longus, and iliopsoas, with normal findings in the tibialis anterior, medial gastrocnemius, tensor fascia lata, and upper lumbar paraspinals. Myokymic discharges were recorded in the vastus medialis and adductor longus. These findings indicated a long-standing neurogenic process involving the lumbar plexus, and the presence of myokymic discharges in the context of a history of radiation, increased the suspicion for a radiation-induced upper lumbar plexopathy. If the patient had a history of radiation to midline structures (ie, abdomen or pelvis), needle examination of the contralateral side would have been considered to identify subclinical involvement.

Radiation plexopathies and malignant plexus infiltration may co-exist.[22] In neoplastic lumbosacral plexopathies, pain is more common and is an early presenting symptom, and lymphedema may be present. Malignant plexus invasion is usually identified on MRI; thus, any plexopathy in a patient with a history of cancer should be accompanied by contrast-enhanced imaging.[40] Plexopathies due to radiation injury are more common in doses greater than 5000 cGy but have been reported at lower doses, present years after radiation, are usually slowly progressive, and may demonstrate myokymic discharges on needle electromyography (EMG).

SUMMARY

Evaluation of brachial and lumbosacral plexopathies in the EMG laboratory is challenging. Knowledge of the plexus anatomy, correlation of plexus segments with common and uncommon NCS and the muscles examined during needle EMG, and understanding the anatomic structures that surround the brachial and lumbosacral plexus help to inform the clinician about potential localization and mechanisms of injury and facilitate timely diagnoses. A thorough, systematic EDX approach to plexopathies can assist in the assessment of these complex structures.

CLINICS CARE POINTS

- Plexopathies may be traumatic (i.e., blunt or traction injury), inflammatory (i.e., hereditary or idiopathic plexitis, structural (i.e., malignant infiltration, cervical rib), toxic (i.e., radiation-induced) or vascular (i.e., thromboembolism, vasculitis). Allow a thorough history, examination clues (i.e., presence of a Horner's sign) and imaging studies to guide assessment of the underlying etiology. The presence of pain favours an inflammatory or neoplastic process, and often presents with contrast enhancing neural components on MRI studies. Radiation-induced plexopathies may be painless or with milder discomfort and typically lack the aggressive, enhancing radiographic abnormalities typical of a neoplastic process. Patients in whom a malignancy is highly suspected may require serial imaging for diagnostic confirmation.

- Poor prognostic factors in a traumatic plexopathy include proximal trunk injuries, panplexopathies, presence of concomitant nerve root avulsion, and dense weakness with EDX evidence of poor reinnervation (i.e., low amplitude CMAP, dense fibrillation potentials and minimal MUP activation without nascent units) 4-6 months from the time of injury.

- The main differentiating factor between a very proximal plexopathy (i.e., trunk) and a radiculopathy is an abnormal SNAP. The needle examination will be largely the same in both situations, as examination of paraspinal muscles can in many cases be suboptimal and may not confidently exclude a radiculopathy. This highlights the importance of non-routine sensory studies (i.e., medial antebrachial cutaneous) in definitively assessing a plexopathy.

- A baseline EDX study may be useful in the early days after onset of symptoms. While fibrillation potentials and neurogenic motor units will take weeks to manifest, abnormalities in sensory and motor conduction studies will be readily apparent, as will reduced recruitment of motor units on needle examination. This allows for a timelier diagnosis of etiologies requiring urgent intervention and will highlight any pre-existing, chronic neurogenic processes that may confound the evaluation. A repeat study in 4-6 weeks may be indicated in patients receiving early EDX studies.

- The microvasculitic plexopathy associated with diabetics typically involves the lumbosacral plexus and is accompanied by exquisite pain. Less common presentations, however, have been described and include involvement of the brachial plexus, presentation without pain, lumbosacral plexopathies in non-diabetics, and sequential involvement of the contralateral limb. Be mindful that not all patients will present classically, and a subacute, often painful plexopathy associated with atrophy and weight loss (barring exclusion of infection and malignancy) is often inflammatory in nature and requires prompt initiation of steroids. The underlying pathological process is considered similar in patients with post-surgical inflammatory plexopathies.

DISCLOSURE

The author has nothing to disclose.

REFERENCES

1. Suarez GA, Giannini C, Bosch EP, et al. Immune brachial plexus neuropathy: Suggestive evidence for an inflammatory-immune pathogenesis. Neurology 1996;46(2):559–61.
2. Rubin DI. Brachial and lumbosacral plexopathies: A review. Clin Neurophysiol Pract 2020;5:173–93.
3. Laughlin RS, Dyck PJB. Electrodiagnostic testing in lumbosacral plexopathies. Phys Med Rehabil Clin N Am 2013;24(1):93–105.
4. Chhetri SK, Lekwuwa G, Seriki D, et al. Acute flaccid paraparesis secondary to bilateral ischaemic lumbosacral plexopathy. QJM Mon J Assoc Physicians 2013;106(5):463–5.
5. Dyck PJB, Windebank AJ. Diabetic and nondiabetic lumbosacral radiculoplexus neuropathies: New insights into pathophysiology and treatment. Muscle Nerve 2002;25(4):477–91.
6. Preston DC, Shapiro BE. Brachial plexopathy. In: Electromyography and neuromuscular disorders. 2nd edition. Philadelphia, PA: Elsevier; 2005. p. 479–500.
7. Ferrante MA, Wilbourn AJ. The utility of various sensory nerve conduction responses in assessing brachial plexopathies. Muscle Nerve 1995;18(8):879.
8. Soto O. Radiation-induced conduction block: Resolution following anticoagulant therapy. Muscle Nerve 2005;31(5):642–5.
9. Daube JR, Rubin DI. Needle electromyography. Muscle Nerve 2009;39(2): 244–70.
10. Impastato DM, Impastato KA, Dabestani P, et al. Prognostic value of needle electromyography in traumatic brachial plexus injury. Muscle Nerve 2019;60(5): 595–7.
11. Katirji B, Wilbourn AJ, Scarberry SL, et al. Intrapartum maternal lumbosacral plexopathy. Muscle Nerve 2002;26(3):340–7.
12. Krarup C, Crone C. Neurophysiological studies in malignant disease with particular reference to involvement of peripheral nerves. J Neurol 2002;249(6):651–61.
13. Pham M, Bäumer P, Meinck H-M, et al. Anterior interosseous nerve syndrome: Fascicular motor lesions of median nerve trunk. Neurol 2014;82(7):598–606.
14. Rawal A, Yin Q, Roebuck M, et al. Atypical and malignant peripheral nerve-sheath tumors of the brachial plexus: Report of three cases and review of the literature. Microsurg 2006;26(2):80–6.
15. Sherburn EW, Kaplan SS, Kaufman BA, et al. Outcome of surgically treated birth-related brachial plexus injuries in twenty cases. Pediatr Neurosurg 1997;27(1):19.
16. Staff NP, Engelstad J, Klein CJ, et al. Post-surgical inflammatory neuropathy. Brain 2010;133(10):2866–80.
17. Tsao BE, Ostrovskiy DA, Wilbourn AJ, et al. Phrenic neuropathy due to neuralgic amyotrophy. Neurology 2006;66(10):1582–4.
18. Windebank AJ, Schenone A, Dewald GW. Hereditary neuropathy with liability to pressure palsies and inherited brachial plexus neuropathy–two genetically distinct disorders. Mayo Clin Proc 1995;70(8):743.
19. Bertelli MD, PhD JA, Ghizoni MD, et al. Patterns of brachial plexus stretch palsy in a prospective series of 565 surgically treated patients. J Hand Surg Am 2017; 42(6):443–6.e2.
20. Feinberg JH, Nguyen ET, Boachie-Adjei K, et al. The electrodiagnostic natural history of parsonage–turner syndrome. Muscle Nerve 2017;56(4):737–43.
21. Ferrante MA. Electrodiagnostic assessment of the brachial plexus. Neurol Clin 2012;30(2):551–80.

22. Harper CMJ, Thomas JE, Cascino TL, et al. Distinction between neoplastic and radiation-induced brachial plexopathy, with emphasis on the role of EMG. Neurol 1989;39(4):502.

23. Healey S, O'Neill B, Bilal H, et al. Does retraction of the sternum during median sternotomy result in brachial plexus injuries? Interact Cardiovasc Thorac Surg 2013;17(1):151–7.

24. Jaeckle KA. Neurologic manifestations of neoplastic and radiation-induced plexopathies. Semin Neurol 2010;30(3):254–62.

25. Noland SS, Bishop AT, Spinner RJ, et al. Adult traumatic brachial plexus injuries. J Am Acad Orthop Surg 2019;27(19):705–16.

26. Sánchez-Soblechero A, García CA, Sáez Ansotegui A, et al. Upper trunk brachial plexopathy as a consequence of prone positioning due to SARS-CoV-2 acute respiratory distress syndrome. Muscle Nerve 2020;62(5):E76–8.

27. Feinberg J. EMG: Myths and facts. HSS J 2006;2(1):19–21.

28. Spinner RJ, Kline DG. Surgery for peripheral nerve and brachial plexus injuries or other nerve lesions. Muscle Nerve 2000;23(5):680–95.

29. Parsonage MJ, Aldren Turner JW. Neuralgic amyotrophy: the shouldergirdle syndrome. Lancet 1948;251(6513):973–8.

30. Tsairis P, Dyck PJ, Mulder DW. Natural history of brachial plexus neuropathy: Report on 99 patients. Arch Neurol 1972;27(2):109–17.

31. Ferrante MA. The thoracic outlet syndromes. Muscle Nerve 2012;45(6):780–95.

32. Tsao BE, Ferrante MA, Wilbourn AJ, et al. Electrodiagnostic features of true neurogenic thoracic outlet syndrome. Muscle Nerve 2014;49(5):724–7.

33. Bourque PR, Warman Chardon J, Bryanton M, et al. Neurolymphomatosis of the brachial plexus and its branches: case series and literature review. Can J Neurol Sci 2018;45(2):137–43.

34. Ko K, Sung DH, Kang MJ, et al. Clinical, electrophysiological findings in adult patients with non-traumatic plexopathies. Ann Rehabil Med 2011;35(6):807.

35. Preston DC, Shapiro BE. Lumbosacral plexopathy. In: Electromyography and neuromuscular disorders. 2nd edition. Elsevier; 2005. p. 517–35.

36. Abel NA, Abel NA, Januszewski J, et al. Femoral nerve and lumbar plexus injury after minimally invasive lateral retroperitoneal transpsoas approach: electrodiagnostic prognostic indicators and a roadmap to recovery. Neurosurg Rev 2018; 41(2):457–64.

37. Kutsy RL, Robinson LR, Routt ML. Lumbosacral plexopathy in pelvic trauma. Muscle Nerve 2000;23(11):1757–60.

38. Czyrny JJ, Lawrence J. The importance of paraspinal muscle EMG in cervical and lumbosacral radiculopathy: review of 100 cases. Electromyogr Clin Neurophysiol 1996;36(8):503.

39. Katirji B, Wilbourn AJ. High sciatic lesion mimicking peroneal neuropathy at the fibular head. J Neurol Sci 1994;121(2):172–5.

40. Capek S, Howe BM, Amrami KK, et al. Perineural spread of pelvic malignancies to the lumbosacral plexus and beyond: clinical and imaging patterns. Neurosurg Focus 2015;39(3):E14.

Electrodiagnostic Assessment of Polyneuropathy

Rocio Vazquez Do Campo, MD*

KEYWORDS

- Polyneuropathy • Nerve conduction studies • Needle electromyography
- Axonal neuropathy • Demyelinating neuropathy • Nodopathy • Paranodopathy
- Conduction block

KEY POINTS

- Nerve conduction studies and needle electromyography, collectively known as electrodiagnostic (EDX) studies, are a sensitive and objective method to assess the function and integrity of peripheral nerves.
- Despite recent advances in other areas, such as laboratory, genetic testing, or peripheral nerve imaging techniques, EDX studies remain the "gold standard" for the diagnosis, quantification, and classification of polyneuropathies.
- One of the main goals of the EDX evaluation is to classify polyneuropathies into primary *axonal* or *demyelinating*. Recently, a third group of neuropathies characterized by impaired conduction at the nodes of Ranvier, *nodo-paranodopathies*, has been described.
- Electrophysiological techniques and protocols for the evaluation of polyneuropathy vary greatly among neurophysiology laboratories. More efforts toward standardization are required to improve the reproducibility of EDX testing and facilitate epidemiologic and research studies.

INTRODUCTION

Peripheral neuropathies, or polyneuropathies, are a heterogeneous group of inherited and acquired disorders with a relatively high prevalence in the general population and for which hundreds of potential etiologies have been identified. Peripheral neuropathies result from widespread damage to peripheral nerves and cause various degrees of sensory, motor, and autonomic dysfunction depending on the severity and type of nerve fibers involved. The clinical diagnosis of polyneuropathy relies heavily on pattern recognition, which takes into account: functional modalities affected, anatomic distribution of symptoms and signs, temporal course, patient's risk factors, family history and accompanying systemic manifestations.

Department of Neurology, University of Alabama at Birmingham, 260 Sparks Center, 1720 7th Avenue S, Birmingham, AL 35294, USA
* Corresponding author.
E-mail address: rcampo@uabmc.edu

Neurol Clin 39 (2021) 1015–1034
https://doi.org/10.1016/j.ncl.2021.06.012
0733-8619/21/© 2021 Elsevier Inc. All rights reserved.

Determining whether small or large nerve fibers are predominantly affected is often possible through careful review of the patient's symptoms and a thorough neurologic examination, including testing of all modalities of sensation (vibration, joint position, light touch, temperature, and pain), motor examination, and reflexes (**Table 1**). The identification of small versus large fiber-type predilection helps narrow the differential diagnosis and direct subsequent investigations, including most appropriate neurophysiological tests, laboratory studies, and, in some cases, most adequate tissue biopsy (nerve or skin) or genetic testing. Routine electrodiagnostic (EDX) studies assess the population of large myelinated sensory and motor fibers only. The diagnosis of pure small fiber neuropathy requires other investigations, such as assessment of intraepidermal nerve fiber density or testing of autonomic functions.

GENERAL CONSIDERATIONS
What Information Can Be Obtained from EDX Studies?

As polyneuropathy symptoms can mimic other neurologic or non-neurologic conditions (eg, bilateral lumbosacral radiculopathies, plantar fasciitis) and examination findings are often mild or subjective, EDX studies provide objective information that complements the clinical evaluation and helps confirm or exclude the presence of polyneuropathy (**Box 1**).

Are EDX Studies Required in All Patients?

Universal EDX testing in patients with a clinical suspicion of polyneuropathy is controversial.[1-3] Some studies suggest limited diagnostic utility and poor cost-effectiveness in mild distal predominantly sensory polyneuropathy when the cause is suspected (eg, diabetes) and results are not expected to influence management decisions.[1,3] On the contrary, EDX evaluation should be strongly considered in patients with moderate/severe symptoms, acute/subacute presentation, atypical features (motor predominance, proximal or asymmetric deficits, diffuse sensory loss or marked ataxia), foot deformities (high arches, hammertoes) and/or family history of polyneuropathy, or if the etiology remains uncertain despite other investigations.[3] Understanding the pathophysiology, severity, and chronicity of the neuropathy is important to provide adequate counseling and establish prognosis.

What Are the Components of the EDX Evaluation of Polyneuropathy?

Sensory and motor nerve conduction studies

Routine sensory and motor nerve conduction studies (NCS) are obtained from stimulation and recording over distal limb segments; therefore, they are quite sensitive to detect pathologic changes in polyneuropathy. Most polyneuropathies are characterized by "dying-back" axonal degeneration and demonstrate earlier and more prominent abnormalities in NCS obtained from the lower limbs. Sensory fibers, which are more susceptible to toxic and metabolic insults, are often affected first and, as the severity of the polyneuropathy increases, motor fibers and nerves in the upper limbs become involved.

NCS yield 2 types of measures of integrity and function of axons and myelin, respectively: the amplitude of the evoked response and parameters that reflect velocity of nerve conduction. Abnormalities on parameters of nerve conduction, which include distal latency (DL), F-wave latency, and conduction velocity (CV), are reliable indicators of peripheral nerve disease. Reduced compound motor action potential (CMAP) amplitudes can be observed in other neurogenic and non-neurogenic disorders, including lower motor neuron disease or myopathies, and are less specific for peripheral nerve localization. Reduced sensory nerve action potential (SNAP) amplitudes

Table 1
Small and large fiber (sensory and motor predominant) polyneuropathies: clinical and examination features, associated disorders, and neurophysiological tests

	Small Fiber	Large fiber (sensory)	Large fiber (motor)
Symptoms	**Positive:** Prickling, stabbing, lancinating or electrical shock-like pain, thermal dysesthesias (burning pain or coldness) **Negative:** numbness, reduced sensation for hot and cold temperatures **Autonomic:** dry eyes, dry mouth, palpitations, orthostatic lightheadedness, sweating abnormalities, early satiety, constipation, urinary retention, erectile dysfunction	**Positive:** tingling, "buzzing" sensation **Negative:** numbness, imbalance, reduced coordination, and dexterity	**Positive:** cramping, fasciculations (less common) **Negative:** weakness
Examination findings	Hypo- or anesthesia to pinprick, temperature and light touch, hyperalgesia to pinprick, contact allodynia, dry skin, foot discoloration. Normal strength, reflexes, joint position, and vibration	Reduced joint position and vibration; altered tandem gait, limb ataxia, hyporeflexia or areflexia. Absent or mild weakness	Weakness and muscle atrophy; hyporeflexia or areflexia. Milder sensory deficits
Associated disorders	Diabetes, obesity and metabolic syndrome, alcoholism, uremia, Sjögren syndrome and other connective tissue disorders, hepatitis C and HIV infection, amyloidosis (AL and transthyretin), sarcoidosis. Fabry disease, Tangier disease, hereditary sensory and autonomic neuropathy, sodium channelopathies (SCN9A, SCN10A, SCN11A mutations)	Diabetes, end-stage renal disease, inherited, vitamin deficiencies (B12, thiamine), vitamin B6 toxicity, Sjögren syndrome, paraneoplastic, HIV infection, chemotherapy-induced, DADS neuropathy, sensory CIDP and CISP, Miller-Fisher syndrome	CIDP, Guillain-Barré syndrome, multifocal motor neuropathy, POEMS syndrome, vasculitis, transthyretin amyloidosis, Charcot-Marie-Tooth disease, hereditary neuropathy with liability to pressure palsies, acute intermittent porphyria

(continued on next page)

	Small Fiber	Large fiber (sensory)	Large fiber (motor)
Table 1 (continued)			
Neurophysiological tests	Quantitative sensory testing, thermoregulatory sweat test, autonomic reflex screen (QSART, heart rate to deep breathing, Valsalva, tilt table)	NCS and needle EMG Other: somatosensory evoked potentials and blink reflexes	NCS and needle EMG Other: blink reflexes

Abbreviations: AL, amyloid light-chain; DADS, distal acquired demyelinating symmetric; HIV, human immunodeficiency virus; POEMS, polyneuropathy organomegaly endocrinopathy monoclonal protein and skin changes; QSART, quantitative sudomotor axon reflex test.

indicate the disease is located at or distal to the dorsal root ganglion, whereas normal SNAPs are expected in preganglionic lesions (eg, polyradiculopathy).

F-waves

The advantage of F-waves over conventional motor NCS is that conduction along the entire motor nerve, including proximal segments, can be evaluated. Owing to longer recording distances, F-waves may accentuate mild generalized slowing and be an early indicator of polyneuropathy. The study of F-waves is also useful to establish the proximal-distal distribution of CV along motor nerves by comparing the F-wave latency with the *F-estimate,* which is calculated assuming CV is the same along the entire length of the nerve: $F_{estimate} = [(2 \times \text{distance from stimulation site to spinal cord})/CV] + DL.$[4] The CV and DL used are those previously obtained during the preceding motor study of the same nerve. When there is disproportionate slowing in proximal nerve segments (eg, polyradiculopathy), F-wave latencies are longer than their estimate.

Needle electromyography

Needle electromyography (EMG) is particularly sensitive to detect changes related to axonal loss (denervation and reinnervation) and can identify motor involvement before it becomes clinically evident (**Box 2**). The distribution and magnitude of fibrillation potentials along with changes in motor unit potential (MUP) morphology and firing pattern are analyzed to determine the chronology and severity of polyneuropathy and the efficacy of reinnervation. Axonal polyneuropathies demonstrate enlarged

---

Box 1
Goals of the electrodiagnostic evaluation in polyneuropathy

- Confirm the presence of large fiber polyneuropathy, detect subclinical abnormalities, and exclude alternative or superimposed neuromuscular conditions. Determine the type of nerve fibers involved (sensory, motor or both), and the chronology (acute, subacute or chronic) and severity of nerve damage. Identify the underlying pathophysiological process (primary axonal or demyelinating). Establish the anatomic distribution of nerve involvement (length-dependent or non–length-dependent; diffuse, focal, or multifocal)

- Monitor for worsening, improvement or stability of the polyneuropathy over time. Monitor response to therapeutic interventions

---

Box 2
Role of needle electromyography in polyneuropathy

- Detect and quantify severity of denervation (fibrillation potentials).
- Assess chronicity of axonal injury and efficacy of reinnervation (changes in motor unit potential morphology: polyphasia, instability, increased duration and amplitude).
- Evaluate motor unit recruitment pattern in axonal and demyelinating neuropathies.
- Localize and evaluate extent of nerve injury (anatomic distribution of muscle findings).
- Identify other spontaneous discharges (fasciculations, myotonia, neuromyotonia, complex repetitive discharges).

---

and complex MUPs with or without fibrillation potentials, whereas reduced recruitment of MUPs out of proportion to denervation and reinnervation changes is characteristic of demyelinating neuropathies. One of the most important roles of needle EMG is to evaluate the extent and site of nerve injury based on the anatomic distribution of muscles involved. A distal-to-proximal gradient of abnormalities is typically observed in length-dependent polyneuropathies, while diffuse involvement of proximal and distal limb and paraspinal muscles suggests a polyradicular pattern.

Other studies
Blink reflex. Although not routinely performed, blink studies may have a role in the evaluation of demyelinating neuropathies and sensory ganglionopathies.[5] Prolonged blink latencies are observed in some acquired and inherited demyelinating neuropathies, whereas most axonal polyneuropathies demonstrate normal blink responses.[5,6] Blink studies can be considered when conventional NCS are equivocal for demyelination or limb responses are absent or markedly low, precluding adequate assessment of CVs. In addition, blink reflexes are frequently normal in paraneoplastic sensory ganglionopathies (eg, ANNA-1), but may demonstrate absent/delayed R1 responses with or without R2 abnormalities in nonparaneoplastic sensory ganglionopathies (eg, Sjogren's syndrome).[7]

Somatosensory evoked potentials. Somatosensory evoked potentials (SEPs) assess conduction along peripheral and central somatosensory pathways and should be considered in patients with sensory disturbances not explained by NCS or spinal cord imaging findings. SEPs can provide evidence of demyelination at the plexus or root level in sensory predominant polyradiculopathies, including sensory variants of Guillain-Barré syndrome (GBS), and chronic inflammatory demyelinating polyradiculoneuropathy (CIDP). SEPs are an important diagnostic tool in chronic immune sensory polyradiculopathy (CISP), a pure sensory variant of CIDP characterized by progressive sensory loss and ataxia. Owing to selective sensory root demyelination and lack of motor involvement, routine EDX studies are normal in CISP and SEPs typically demonstrate delayed lumbar and cervical evoked responses.[8]

PLANNING AND INTERPRETATION OF THE EDX STUDY

One of the most challenging aspects of the EDX evaluation of polyneuropathy is the lack of consensus regarding the most appropriate EDX techniques, set-up protocols, reference values, and number and selection of nerves and muscles to test. A proposed algorithm for the EDX evaluation of polyneuropathy is presented in **Fig. 1**. In general, NCS and needle EMG are performed on one side unless symptoms are asymmetric or

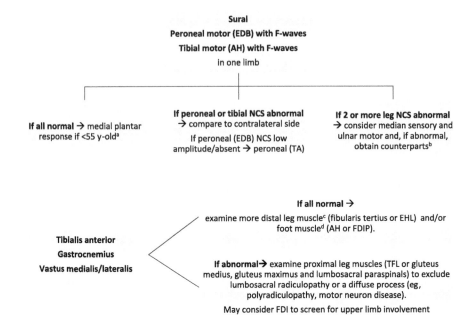

Sural
Peroneal motor (EDB) with F-waves
Tibial motor (AH) with F-waves
in one limb

If all normal → medial plantar response if <55 y-old[a]

If peroneal or tibial NCS abnormal → compare to contralateral side
If peroneal (EDB) NCS low amplitude/absent → peroneal (TA)

If 2 or more leg NCS abnormal → consider median sensory and ulnar motor and, if abnormal, obtain counterparts[b]

Tibialis anterior
Gastrocnemius
Vastus medialis/lateralis

If all normal →
examine more distal leg muscle[c] (fibularis tertius or EHL) and/or foot muscle[d] (AH or FDIP).

If abnormal→ examine proximal leg muscles (TFL or gluteus medius, gluteus maximus and lumbosacral paraspinals) to exclude lumbosacral radiculopathy or a diffuse process (eg, polyradiculopathy, motor neuron disease).
May consider FDI to screen for upper limb involvement

Fig. 1. Proposed NCS (above) and needle EMG (below) algorithm in polyneuropathy. AH, abductor hallucis; EDB, extensor digitorum brevis; EHL, extensor hallucis longus; FDI, first dorsal interosseous; FDIP, first dorsal interosseous pedis; NCS, nerve conduction studies; TA, tibialis anterior; TFL, tensor fascia lata. [a]Medial plantar response evaluation may increase the diagnostic yield for identifying mild distal symmetric polyneuropathy in individuals younger than 55 years. [b]Upper limb NCS should also be performed if: lower limb responses are absent, axonal versus demyelinating classification is not possible based on lower limb NCS only or when predominant upper limb involvement is suspected (eg, immune-mediated neuropathy). [c]Needle examination of fibularis tertius or EHL can be particularly helpful when NCS are normal/mildly abnormal and calf muscles do not yield abnormalities. [d]Fibrillation potentials and reinnervation changes in foot muscles should be interpreted with caution (foot trauma).

to establish side-to-side comparison when responses on one side are absent or low. In neuropathies with patchy or multifocal involvement (eg, mononeuropathy multiplex) testing multiple limbs is recommended. Performing additional studies may increase the diagnostic yield in some situations (eg, additional sensory studies to demonstrate diffuse sensory involvement in a sensory ganglionopathy).

The electrophysiological data must be analyzed in conjunction with the available clinical information. A low threshold to consider and correct potential technical errors should be maintained throughout the study, especially when results are unexpected or inconsistent with the physical examination. Sensory NCS are particularly prone to technical and interpretative errors. Owing to their low amplitude (microvolts), anatomic variation among individuals and susceptibility to technical and age-related factors, lower limb SNAPs may be difficult to obtain and absent responses without clinical correlation should be interpreted with caution.[9,10] In addition, background noise and random baseline variations should not be mistaken for "true" SNAPs and averaging of several traces is recommended to demonstrate accuracy and consistency of the responses.[10] In the upper limbs, focal entrapment neuropathies should be excluded before abnormal median and ulnar SNAPs can be attributed to polyneuropathy.

Variables such as temperature, patient's age, body mass index, or height can influence parameters of the test and must be taken into account.[10]

PATHOPHYSIOLOGY OF NERVE INJURY: AXONAL LOSS, DEMYELINATION, AND NODO-PARANODAL DYSFUNCTION

One of the main goals of the EDX evaluation is to classify polyneuropathies into *axonal* or *demyelinating* based on the primary mechanism of nerve injury. Recently, a third group of neuropathies, *nodo-paranodopathies*, has been described. Nodo-paranodopathies are neither primary axonal nor demyelinating, but rather characterized by impaired conduction at the nodes of Ranvier, which may be transitory and reversible with prompt recovery or progress to axonal degeneration with worse outcomes.[11,12]

Axonal Loss

Axonal degeneration is the most common pathologic substrate in peripheral nerve disorders and results from injury to the axon itself (axonopathy) or damage to the cell body of sensory or motor neurons (neuronopathy). Axonal polyneuropathies are characterized by reduced SNAP and CMAP amplitudes, which reflect the loss of sensory and motor axons (and muscle fibers innervated by them), respectively. SNAP amplitudes are especially sensitive to axonal loss because of lack of compensatory collateral reinnervation and are usually affected earlier in polyneuropathies. CMAP amplitudes can be maintained until greater than 80% of axons are lost by means of collateral sprouting and muscle fiber reinnervation.

CV, DL, and F-wave latency may be normal or mildly affected in axonal polyneuropathies, the latter owing to the loss of faster-conducting axons. As a general rule, CV does not drop below 70% of the lower limit of normal (LLN) and DL and F-wave latency do not increase above 125% to 130% of the upper limit of normal (ULN) solely due to axonal loss. This phenomenon, known as *amplitude-dependent* CV slowing, should be considered when interpreting parameters of nerve conduction in the presence of reduced amplitude responses. The electrophysiological features of axonal polyneuropathies are summarized in **Box 3**.

Demyelination

Myelin damage or dysfunction impair saltatory conduction and rapid propagation of action potentials along the axon resulting in CV slowing and even failure of conduction

---

Box 3
Electrophysiological features of axonal polyneuropathies

- Reduced sensory nerve and compound muscle action potential amplitudes.
- Conduction velocity normal or mildly decreased, but remains >70% of the lower limit of normal.
- Distal latency and F-wave latency normal or mildly prolonged, but remain <125 to 130% of the upper limit of normal.
- No temporal dispersion or conduction block.
- Needle electromyography: various degrees of denervation (fibrillation potentials) and reinnervation (long duration, high amplitude, polyphasic motor unit potentials) depending on chronicity and severity.

if severe. Electrophysiological features indicative of demyelination are summarized in **Box 4**.

CV slowing
The most common manifestation of demyelination is marked CV slowing with relative preservation of CMAP and SNAP amplitudes. The degree of CV slowing required to meet criteria for demyelination varies depending on the CMAP amplitude and is at least 70% of the LLN (equivalent to <35 m/s in the arm and <28 m/s in the leg) if the CMAP amplitude is normal and ≤50% of the LLN if the CMAP amplitude is markedly reduced (≤50% of the LLN).

The pattern of CV slowing can help distinguish acquired from inherited demyelinating neuropathies. In acquired disorders, NCS demonstrate different degrees of CV slowing between nerves and segments within a nerve (*nonuniform* slowing), the latter represented by temporal dispersion or conduction block (CB), because of the multifocal and segmental distribution of demyelination. On the contrary, all nerves show a similar degree of CV slowing (*uniform* slowing) in most inherited demyelinating neuropathies due to myelin abnormalities present along the entire length of the nerve.

DL and F-wave latency prolongation
DL and F-wave latency are good measures of conduction over distal and proximal nerve segments, respectively, and may be significantly prolonged in demyelinating neuropathies. The degree of DL or F-wave latency prolongation indicative of demyelination ranges between 130% and 150% of the ULN, depending on the criteria used.[13,14] Other F-wave abnormalities that may suggest demyelination include absence or decreased persistence of F waves when the distal CMAP amplitude is preserved (suggesting block of conduction proximally) and increased chronodispersion (latency difference between the shortest and the longest F-wave latency values). It should be noted that F-waves can be absent or prolonged when distal CMAPs are markedly reduced due to axonal loss (not to be mistaken for demyelination) and in focal disorders that cause nerve root demyelination, such as compressive radiculopathies.

The terminal latency index estimates the degree of CV slowing in distal nerve segments and can be calculated for motor nerves using the formula: (1/distal motor latency) × (distal distance/motor CV). A terminal latency index below 0.25 indicates

---

Box 4
Electrophysiological features of demyelinating polyneuropathies

- Conduction velocity <70% of the lower limit of normal (LLN) (<50% if compound muscle action potential amplitude <50% of the LLN)
- Distal latency >150% of the upper limit of normal (ULN)
- F-wave latency >130% of the ULN
- Prolonged blink latency (R1 >13 milliseconds)
- Temporal dispersion and/or motor conduction block [a]
- Needle electromyography: no fibrillation potentials (or minimal) in pure demyelinating process; reduced recruitment of motor unit potentials out of proportion to denervation and reinnervation changes

[a]Typical of acquired demyelinating neuropathies and rare in hereditary demyelinating neuropathies.

more prominent demyelination in distal nerve segments and is typically observed in neuropathies associated with Ig M paraproteinemias.[15]

Increased temporal dispersion

Temporal dispersion reflects variability of CV among different axons with action potentials arriving at the recording electrodes at slightly different times, resulting in increased duration of the recorded response. Given that some degree of physiologic temporal dispersion occurs in sensory axons, abnormal temporal dispersion is more reliably assessed in motor axons. Abnormal temporal dispersion is defined as an increase of the negative CMAP duration, measured from the onset to the end of the negative component of the response, greater than 30% with proximal compared with distal stimulation. Abnormally dispersed responses exhibit an asynchronous and irregularly contoured morphology and represent multifocal demyelination along the studied nerve segment (**Fig. 2**).

Conduction block

CB refers to the failure of an action potential to propagate along a structurally intact axon. The underlying pathophysiology may represent focal demyelination at the internodes or functional disturbance at the nodes of Ranvier. CB is defined by a larger negative CMAP area (or amplitude) when a nerve is stimulated distal compared with proximal to the site of block. The proximal CMAP duration should not increase more than 30% to exclude superimposed temporal dispersion over the same nerve segment (**Fig. 3**).

The criteria for *definite* CB vary among different nerves and is defined as a negative CMAP area reduction between distal and proximal stimulation greater than 50% for the median, ulnar, and fibular nerves (**Box 5**).[16] The *minimal* criteria for CB in most nerves is defined as a CMAP area reduction greater than 20%, except for the tibial nerve in which up to a 50% reduction is considered normal. It is important to note that CB in distal nerve segments may result in reduced distal CMAP amplitude mimicking an axonal process. Also, when distal CMAP amplitudes are significantly reduced (<1 mV or <20% of the LLN), the presence of CB in proximal nerve segments cannot be reliably established. CB correlates with reduced recruitment of MUPs and is often proportional to the degree of muscle weakness observed on examination.

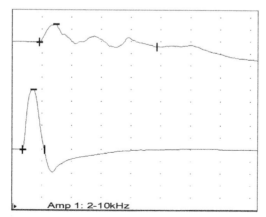

Fig. 2. Temporal dispersion in the median motor nerve (recording over the abductor pollicis brevis). Note the amplitude drop from the wrist (10 mV) to the elbow (3.1 mV) and the abnormally dispersed at the elbow.

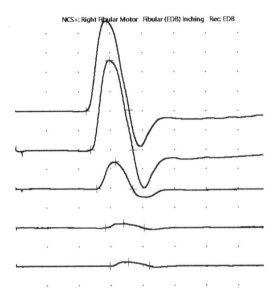

NCS+: Right Fibular Motor Fibular (EDB) Inching Rec: EDB

Fig. 3. Conduction block in the peroneal (fibular) nerve across the fibular head demonstrating amplitude drop (from 9.3 to 0.44 mV) without increase in response duration.

Mixed Pattern: Axonal Loss with Disproportionate CV Slowing

Some neuropathies demonstrate reduced CMAP and SNAP amplitudes with a moderate degree of CV slowing that does not meet criteria for primary demyelination. This pattern is commonly observed in polyneuropathies associated with diabetes and end-stage renal disease in which axonal membrane dysfunction due to metabolic factors may accentuate CV slowing out of proportion to amplitude changes (*amplitude-independent* CV slowing), particularly in the lower limbs.[14,17] Even asymptomatic

---

Box 5
Electrophysiological criteria for motor conduction block

Definite:[a]
- >50% negative CMAP area reduction with proximal vs distal stimulation of median, ulnar, or fibular (peroneal) nerve.
- Negative distal CMAP amplitude must be >20% of the lower limit of normal and >1 mV, AND
- Increase of proximal negative peak CMAP duration must be ≤ 30%.

Probable:[a]
- ≥30% negative CMAP area reduction with proximal vs distal stimulation of upper limb nerve with an increase of proximal to distal negative peak CMAP duration ≤30%, OR
- ≥50% negative CMAP area reduction (same as definite) with an increase of proximal to distal negative peak CMAP duration >30%

[a]Evidence of conduction block must be found at sites distinct from common entrapment or compression syndromes.

Adapted from: European Federation of Neurological Societies/Peripheral Nerve Society Guideline on management of multifocal motor neuropathy. Report of a Joint Task Force of the European Federation of Neurological Societies and the Peripheral Nerve Society – first revision. J Peripher Nerv Syst 2010;15:295-301; with permission.

diabetic patients can have CVs in the LLN with preserved amplitudes. To avoid over-estimation of the demyelinating component and errors in interpretation, strict adherence to demyelinating criteria and clinical judgment are strongly encouraged. A length-dependent pattern of symptoms, signs, and chronic reinnervation changes on EMG favors diabetic neuropathy over demyelinating polyradiculoneuropathies, such as CIDP.

Nodo-paranodal dysfunction

The classic dichotomous classification of polyneuropathies into axonal and demyelinating subtypes has been defined by the emergence of a new concept, nodo-paranodopathy. Dysfunction or disruption of gangliosides, axo-glial proteins (contactin-1, neurofascin-155), and ion channels that maintain structural integrity and function of the nodes of Ranvier and paranodal regions have been proposed as a third type of nerve injury.[11,18]

Nodopathies and paranodopathies are characterized by a pathophysiological *continuum* initiated by disruption of conduction at the nodes of Ranvier, which may be potentially reversible in early stages (*reversible conduction failure*), or may be followed by microstructural (myelin detachment, node lengthening) and electrophysiological (sodium channel dysfunction, abnormal membrane polarization) alterations, eventually leading to axonal degeneration.[11] Nodo-paranodal dysfunction has been described in neuropathies associated with immune-mediated and energy restriction mechanisms, the latter including toxic, nutritional, or ischemic (**Box 6**).[12]

It has been proposed that, to capture the different pathophysiological stages of nodo-paranodopathies and detect reversible conduction failure, serial EDX evaluations are required. Early on, NCS demonstrate reduced SNAP and CMAP amplitudes because of nodal conduction failure in distal nerve segments, mimicking an axonal process. CV slowing and DL prolongation, even in the demyelinating range, may be observed possibly due to increased time for action potential propagation at each node. If conduction at the nodes is restored quickly, patients experience prompt recovery and subsequent studies show a rapid increase in SNAP and CMAP amplitudes and DL normalization without the development of excessive temporal dispersion (as it would be expected with remyelination after demyelination). If not reversed, nodal dysfunction triggers a cascade of events leading to axonal degeneration with EDX studies eventually demonstrating typical axonal features.[12,18]

Box 6
Nodo-paranodopathies

- Axonal variants of Guillain-Barré syndrome (AMAN, AMSAN, ASAN).
- CIDP associated with antibodies to nodal and paranodal antigens (neurofascin-186, neurofascin-155, contactin-1, and CASPR1).
- Miller Fisher syndrome.
- Multifocal motor neuropathy.
- Possibly critical illness, ischemic and thiamine deficiency related polyneuropathies.

ASAN, acute sensory ataxic neuropathy; CASPR1, contactin-associated protein 1.

Data from: Uncini A, Santoro L. The electrophysiology of axonal neuropathies: more than just evidence of axonal loss. Clin Neurophysiol 2020;131:2367-74.

DEFINING THE SEVERITY OF POLYNEUROPATHY

There is no universally accepted EDX classification to establish the severity of poly-neuropathy. Furthermore, the severity of the electrophysiological findings does not always correlate with the severity of the patient's symptoms. In axonal polyneuropathies, the number and distribution of nerves and muscles involved, the degree of amplitude reduction, and the magnitude of denervation and reinnervation changes can provide a general overview of severity. An axonal polyneuropathy can be considered mild if only sensory responses in the leg are abnormal and severe if CMAPs and SNAPs are diffusely absent and severe denervation and incomplete rein-nervation are encountered. In demyelinating neuropathies, the number of affected nerves and the magnitude of CB and reduced recruitment correlate better with the degree of weakness than other demyelinating parameters, such as CV slowing or DL prolongation.[19]

MONITORING DISEASE PROGRESSION OR TREATMENT EFFECT

Although not required in most circumstances, follow-up EDX studies can provide an objective measure of the response to therapeutic interventions or the rate of disease progression. The sum of the raw values of the motor and sensory amplitudes—the *summated* CMAPs and *summated* SNAPs, respectively—can be useful to monitor interval changes in both axonal neuropathies and demyelinating neuropathies with secondary axonal loss.[20,21] Ideally, comparison of the summated CMAPs and SNAPs between studies requires testing the same set of motor and sensory nerves using similar techniques and set-up protocols.[22]

The decision to obtain follow-up EDX studies should be individualized and guided by the type of polyneuropathy and the availability and time to the estimated effect of specific treatments. Reexamination can be considered in rapidly evolving (eg, GBS) or relapsing (eg, mononeuropathy multiplex) neuropathies, or when follow-up evaluations are necessary to guide treatment decisions.[23] A 3- to 6-month interval between studies is the minimum recommended after immunotherapy initiation, whereas a 1- to 2-year interval may be more appropriate to monitor slowly progressive poly-neuropathies for which no specific disease-modifying treatments are available.

ELECTROPHYSIOLOGICAL FEATURES OF SELECTED POLYNEUROPATHIES
Distal Symmetric Polyneuropathy

The term distal symmetric polyneuropathy (DSP) defines a group of neuropathies characterized by a symmetric pattern of numbness, tingling, and/or pain with or without weakness that begins in the toes and gradually progresses in a stocking-and-glove pattern. DSP is the most common pattern of polyneuropathy and can be associated with multitude of etiologies, including inherited, toxic-metabolic, nutri-tional, or infectious. The diagnosis of DSP requires a combination of length-dependent neuropathic symptoms and signs along with NCS abnormalities on at least 2 separate nerves, one of which must be the sural.[24,25] **Table 2** summarizes the elec-trophysiological characteristics of polyneuropathies presenting with a distal symmet-ric pattern.

Inherited Polyneuropathies

Charcot-Marie-Tooth (CMT) disease is the most common among the inherited poly-neuropathies and presents with a variety of phenotypes, modes of inheritance, and causative genes. Subclassification of CMT disease based on median motor CV into

Table 2
Distal symmetric polyneuropathy: electrophysiologic characteristics depending on etiology

	Nerve Conduction Studies	Needle EMG	Comments
Diabetes and end-stage renal disease	Axonal sensory > motor; may show mild/moderate CV slowing without temporal dispersion or conduction block	Length-dependent fibrillation potentials and chronic reinnervation	Need to be distinguished from primary demyelinating neuropathies
Vitamin B12 deficiency	Axonal, sensory > motor involvement	May be normal	May be associated with subacute combined degeneration of the spinal cord
Thiamine deficiency	Axonal sensorimotor with normal CV or mild CV slowing	Frequent fibrillation potentials in distal leg muscles in early stages	Suspect in alcoholics, recurrent vomiting, parenteral nutrition, bariatric surgery. May present as a rapid onset polyradiculoneuropathy
Critical illness	Axonal sensorimotor with normal CV or mild CV slowing and increased CMAP duration	Frequent fibrillation potentials in distal leg muscles in early stages	Often associated with myopathy (suspect if proximal weakness and myopathic changes in proximal limb muscles)
Chemotherapy-induced	Axonal, sensory > motor involvement.	May be normal	Dose-dependent and in temporal relationship with initiation of chemotherapy. Frequently improves with discontinuation of the drug.
TTR Amyloidosis	Axonal sensorimotor, may show mild/moderate CV slowing	Length-dependent fibrillation potentials and chronic reinnervation	Neuropathic pain and autonomic dysfunction may be prominent. May present as a polyradiculoneuropathy
Chronic porphyric neuropathy	Axonal sensorimotor. Motor predominant, may have proximal > distal and upper > lower limb involvement during attacks	Prominent denervation during attacks	Variable autonomic involvement and other accompanying symptoms (abdominal pain, encephalopathy)

Abbreviation: TTR, transthyretin.

demyelinating (<35 m/s), intermediate (35–45 m/s), and axonal (>45 m/s) forms has demonstrated utility in predicting underlying genetic abnormalities (**Table 3**).[26] Uniform CV slowing in the demyelinating range without temporal dispersion or CB is observed in CMT types 1, 3, and 4, and distinguish them from acquired demyelinating neuropathies. CMT1X and some dominantly inherited forms have intermediate-range

Table 3
Electrophysiological classification of Charcot-Marie-Tooth disease and genetic associations

	Nerve Conduction Studies	Needle EMG	CMT Subtype	Gene Associations
Demyelinating	Median motor CV < 35 m/s Uniform CV slowing Prolonged R1 latency (>13 milliseconds) No temporal dispersion or conduction block (exceptions may occur)	Reduced recruitment of MUPs and chronic reinnervation	CMT1 (autosomal dominant), CMT3 (autosomal dominant or recessive), CMT4 (autosomal recessive)	PMP22, MPZ, LITAF, EGR2, and NEFL, among others
Intermediate	Median motor CV 35–45 m/s May show temporal dispersion	Reduced recruitment of MUPs and chronic reinnervation	CMT1X (X-linked)	Connexin-32 (GJB1) and MPZ, among others
Axonal	Median motor CV > 45 m/s Reduced SNAP and CMAP amplitudes	Some fibrillation potentials in distal leg muscles and chronic reinnervation	CMT2 (autosomal dominant or recessive)	MFN2, RAB7, TRPV4, and NEFL, among others

Abbreviations: GJB1, gap junction beta 1; LITAF, lipopolysaccharide-induced TNF-factor; MFN2, mitofusin 2; MPZ, myelin protein zero; NEFL, neurofilament light chain; PMP22, peripheral myelin protein 22.

CV slowing, whereas CMT2 demonstrates typical axonal features.[27] Hereditary neuropathy with liability to pressure palsies has a unique electrophysiological pattern characterized by a background polyneuropathy with diffuse CV slowing in nearly all sensory nerves and prolonged distal motor latencies (predominantly in median and fibular nerves) with superimposed motor CV slowing at common entrapment sites.[28]

Guillain-Barré Syndrome

GBS encompasses a group of immune-mediated polyradiculoneuropathies characterized by rapidly progressive ascending paresthesias and weakness achieving a nadir in 2 to 4 weeks. Some patients develop cranial nerve palsies, autonomic instability, and respiratory failure requiring intensive care and mechanical ventilation. Owing to significant symptom overlap, demyelinating and axonal GBS forms are difficult to differentiate on clinical grounds and electrophysiology plays an important role in subtype classification, exclusion of mimickers, and prognostication.[29]

In patients with the classic demyelinating subtype, acute inflammatory demyelinating polyradiculoneuropathy, the sensitivity of NCS to detect multifocal demyelination varies depending on the timing of the study and may be as low as 22% in early stages but increases to 87% at 5 weeks. Prolongation or decreased persistence of F-waves may be the only abnormality in the first week. Another early finding, the *sural sparing* pattern (preservation of the sural response in the presence of abnormal upper limb sensory responses) has been proposed as an element of the GBS EDX criteria.[30] Typical acquired demyelinating features peak at 2 to 3 weeks after onset and may be followed by secondary axonal loss often appearing at 3 to 4 weeks. Persistently low CMAPs and prominent denervation after the acute phase correlate with a worse prognosis.

The two most common axonal GBS subtypes, acute motor axonal neuropathy (AMAN) and acute motor and sensory axonal neuropathy (AMSAN), are presumably caused by an antiganglioside (GM1, GD1a, or GD1b) antibody-mediated attack at the nodes of Ranvier.[12,29] In early stages, AMAN and AMSAN are characterized by marked reduction of amplitudes due to nodal conduction failure/block in distal and intermediate nerve segments, which may be accompanied by CB in more proximal segments and prolonged DLs with some degree of CV slowing. This early "mixed" electrophysiological pattern can lead to diagnostic confusion between axonal and demyelinating GBS subtypes and some experts advocate for a follow-up EDX study within the first 4 to 6 weeks to reach a more accurate diagnosis.[29] Rapid clinical improvement along with normalization of CMAP amplitudes and parameters of CV on follow-up studies supports reversible conduction failure and favors AMAN or AMSAN. However, a significant proportion of patients have persistently low CMAPs and eventually develop secondary axonal degeneration, which renders a worse prognosis.

Miller Fisher syndrome, a less common GBS variant that presents with ataxia, areflexia, ophthalmoparesis, and elevated GQ1b antibodies, demonstrates prominent sensory involvement resembling an axonal neuropathy or neuronopathy with milder demyelinating features and minimal motor involvement.[31]

CIDP and Its Variants

Classic or "typical" CIDP presents with progressive (>8 weeks) symmetric proximal and distal weakness, length-dependent large fiber sensory deficits, and areflexia. The diagnosis of CIDP relies on a combination of clinical features, albuminocytologic dissociation in cerebrospinal fluid, and electrophysiological evidence of segmental demyelination. Several EDX criteria for CIDP have been proposed, all requiring some combination of demyelinating features present in at least 2 motor nerves. The European Federation of Neurological Societies/Peripheral Nerve Society criteria demonstrate high sensitivity (73%–85%) and specificity (91%–95%) for the diagnosis of CIDP and are the most widely used in clinical practice (**Box 7**).[13] "Atypical" CIDP forms may meet definite CIDP electrophysiological criteria but demonstrate distinct clinical and electrophysiological features as shown in **Table 4**.[32]

Despite well-established CIDP EDX criteria, misinterpretation of EDX studies is a common source of diagnostic errors (**Box 8**).[33] CIDP should also be distinguished from the polyneuropathy of POEMS (polyneuropathy, organomegaly, endocrinopathy, monoclonal protein, and skin changes) syndrome. Compared with CIDP, patients with POEMS syndrome demonstrate more uniform demyelination with less temporal dispersion and CB, greater axonal loss with more prominent amplitude reduction and fibrillation potentials, and absent sural sparing.[34]

Multifocal Motor Neuropathy

Multifocal motor neuropathy (MMN) represents a rare, slowly or stepwise progressive, immune-mediated motor neuropathy characterized by asymmetric focal weakness and atrophy in the distribution of one or more individual nerves with absent/minimal sensory disturbances. Upper limb predominance with cramping and fasciculations are common. Up to 40% to 60% of patients have elevated GM1 antibodies.

The hallmark of MMN is the presence of motor CB at noncompressible sites, with normal sensory conduction across the same nerve segment and no temporal dispersion. Criteria sets for MMN require *definite* CB in at least two nerves for definite MMN, and *probable* CB in at least two nerves for probable MMN, along with normal

---

Box 7
EFNS/PNS, European Federation of Neurologic Societies/Peripheral Nerve Society electrodiagnostic criteria for chronic inflammatory demyelinating polyradiculopathy

Definite (at least one of the following):
- Conduction velocity: $\geq$30% reduction below the LLN in 2 nerves.
- Distal motor latency: $\geq$50% above the ULN in 2 nerves (excluding median neuropathy at the wrist from carpal tunnel syndrome).
- F-wave latency: $\geq$30% above the ULN ($\geq$50% if the amplitude of distal CMAP < 80% of LLN) in 2 nerves.
- Absent F waves (if distal CMAP $\geq$20% of LLN) in 2 nerves + one other demyelinating parameter in one other nerve.
- Partial motor conduction block: $\geq$50% CMAP amplitude reduction (if distal CMAP $\geq$20% of LLN) in 2 nerves, OR in 1 nerve + one other demyelinating parameter in one other nerve.
- Abnormal temporal dispersion ($\geq$30% increase in proximal CMAP duration) in 2 nerves.
- Distal CMAP duration increase in 2 nerves (median $\geq$6.6 ms, ulnar $\geq$6.7 ms, peroneal $\geq$7.6 ms, tibial $\geq$8.8 ms) + one other demyelinating parameter in one other nerve.

Probable:
- Partial motor conduction block $\geq$30% (if distal CMAP $\geq$20% of LLN) in 2 nerves, excluding the posterior tibial nerve, OR in 1 nerve + one other demyelinating parameter in one other nerve.

Possible:
- As in definite but in only one nerve.

Adapted from: European Federation of Neurological Societies/Peripheral Nerve Society Guideline on management of chronic inflammatory demyelinating polyradiculoneuropathy: Report of a joint task force of the European Federation of Neurologic Societies and the Peripheral Nerve Society - first revision. Eur J Neurol 2010:17:356-63; with permission.

Table 4
Atypical CIDP variants: clinical and electrophysiologic characteristics

	Clinical Features	Electrophysiology	Comments
Distal CIDP or DADS	Distal and symmetric, sensory > motor, lower > upper limb involvement. Reflexes normal or reduced distally	Disproportionately prolonged distal latencies (TLI ≤0.25), abnormal sural response	Often associated with Ig M monoclonal gammopathy, anti-MAG antibodies in 60% of cases, often refractory to treatment
Multifocal CIDP or MADSAM	Asymmetric motor and sensory, may be upper limb predominant. Reflexes may be normal in the unaffected limb	CV slowing, temporal dispersion, and/or conduction block in affected nerves	Needs to be distinguished from multifocal motor neuropathy
Motor CIDP	Symmetric proximal and distal motor deficits. Reflexes usually reduced	Motor conduction block in multiple nerves, sensory NCS may be abnormal	Rare, good response to IVIG
Sensory CIDP	Pure sensory, may have ataxia. Reflexes globally reduced/absent	Demyelinating motor and sensory NCS	Relatively rare
CISP	Progressive sensory loss and marked ataxia, normal strength. Reflexes globally reduced/absent	Normal NCS and needle EMG	Diagnosis relies on SEPs, CSF analysis, and MRI abnormalities on lumbosacral roots
Antibody-mediated paranodopathies	**Contactin-1 (CNTN1):** Subacute onset, symmetric motor > sensory, sensory ataxia. Nephrotic syndrome in some patients **Neurofascin-155 (NF-155):** Subacute onset, symmetric motor > sensory; may have sensory ataxia and tremor, younger age	More pronounced demyelinating features than typical CIDP; greater CV slowing and motor distal latency and F-wave latency prolongation	Good response to Rituximab and plasma exchange, partial response to corticosteroids, refractory to IVIG. Very high CSF protein in neurofascin-155

Abbreviations: CSF, cerebrospinal fluid; DADS, distal acquired demyelinating symmetric neuropathy; IVIG, intravenous immunoglobulin; MADSAM, multifocal acquired demyelinating sensory and motor neuropathy; MAG, myelin-associated glycoprotein; MRI, magnetic resonance imaging; TLI, terminal latency index.

Box 8
Common pitfalls in CIDP electrodiagnosis

- Amplitude-independent CV slowing in diabetic polyneuropathy.
- Equivocal degrees of CV slowing in axonal polyneuropathies.
- Distal latency prolongation or CV slowing of fibular (peroneal) nerve when amplitude <1 mV.
- Focal CV slowing at common entrapment sites.
- Distal latency prolongation and CV slowing because of cold limb temperatures.
- Mild CV slowing in motor neuron disease.

Data from: Allen JA, Ney J, Lewis RA. Electrodiagnostic errors contribute to chronic inflammatory demyelinating polyneuropathy misdiagnosis. Muscle Nerve 2018;57(4):542-9.

---

sensory NCS (see **Box 5**).[35] The most commonly affected nerves are the median and ulnar nerves in the forearm. A practical approach to MMN involves studying at least 3 motor nerves per arm (median, ulnar, and radial) with stimulation of proximal segments if CB is absent distally. Although once considered a demyelinating neuropathy, there is growing evidence that MMN is better classified as a nodopathy.[11] The prominent denervation in muscles supplied by nerves with CB also suggests that axonal loss is greater than expected with primary demyelination. The absence of sensory involvement or temporal dispersion distinguishes MMN from multifocal acquired demyelinating sensory and motor neuropathy (MADSAM); this distinction is important because treatment with corticosteroids is effective in MADSAM, whereas it can worsen MMN.

Vasculitic Neuropathy

Vasculitic neuropathies result from inflammation of vasa nervorum causing nerve ischemia and can be confined to the peripheral nervous system (nonsystemic) or affect other organs/tissues (systemic). A vasculitic neuropathy should be considered when a patient presents with recurrent painful episodes of sensory and motor deficits in the territory of individual nerves (mononeuropathy multiplex) or, alternatively, with a painful, often asymmetric sensorimotor polyneuropathy.

The approach to vasculitic neuropathies requires testing multiple limbs, including clinically affected nerves and muscles in each limb, with side-to-side comparison to demonstrate asymmetry and multifocality. Significant side-to-side amplitude differences (often >50%), variable involvement of nerves of similar length in the same limb, and lower amplitudes in upper compared with lower limbs not explained by entrapment or radiculopathy are common findings on NCS.[36] Needle EMG shows denervation in the territory of single or multiple nerves often with significant differences between homologous muscles supporting the asymmetric nature of the condition. In severe and chronic cases, or after multiple attacks, the pattern of electrophysiological findings becomes confluent and may resemble an axonal asymmetric polyneuropathy.

CLINICS CARE POINTS

- Polyneuropathies have a wide range of potential etiologies but a narrow spectrum of symptoms with significant clinical overlap.
- Besides improving diagnostic accuracy, the EDX evaluation provides relevant information for the classification and characterization of polyneuropathies, which has important therapeutic and prognostic implications.

- Although EDX testing may not be required in all cases, most patients likely benefit from EDX evaluation.
- Electrophysiological criteria for axonal and demyelinating neuropathies should be carefully considered when interpreting EDX studies to avoid misdiagnosis and ensure adequate management, particularly concerning the use of immunotherapies.

DISCLOSURE

The author has nothing to disclose.

REFERENCES

1. Callaghan BC, Kerber KA, Lisabeth LL, et al. Role of neurologists and diagnostic tests on the management of distal symmetric polyneuropathy. JAMA Neurol 2014; 71:1143–9.
2. Bodofsky EB, Carter GT, England JD. Is electrodiagnostic testing for polyneuropathy overutilized? Muscle Nerve 2017;55(3):301–4.
3. AANEM policy statement on electrodiagnosis for distal symmetric polyneuropathy. Muscle Nerve 2018;57(2):337–9.
4. Jones L, Watson J. Motor nerve conduction studies. In: Rubin DI, Daube JR, editors. Clinical neurophysiology, chapter 17. 4th edition. New York: Oxford University Press; 2016. p. 257–87.
5. Guney F. Blink reflex alterations in various polyneuropathies. In: Hayat G, editor. Peripheral neuropathy - advances in diagnostic and therapeutic approaches. Rijeka, Croatia: IntechOpen; 2012. p. 85–94.
6. Lai YR, Huang CC, Chiu WC, et al. The role of blink reflex R1 latency as an electrophysiological marker in diabetic distal symmetrical polyneuropathy. Clin Neurophysiol 2020;131:34–9.
7. Auger RG, Windebank AJ, Lucchinetti CF, et al. Role of the blink reflex in the evaluation of sensory neuronopathy. Neurology 1999;53(2):407–8.
8. Sinnreich M, Klein CJ, Daube JR, et al. Chronic immune sensory polyradiculopathy: a possibly treatable sensory ataxia. Neurology 2004;63(9):1662–9.
9. Tankisi H, Pugdahl K, Otto M, et al. Misinterpretation of sural nerve conduction studies due to anatomical variation. Clin Neurophysiol 2014;125:2115–21.
10. Dolan C, Bromberg MB. Nerve conduction pitfalls and pearls in the diagnosis of peripheral neuropathies. Semin Neurol 2010;30:436–42.
11. Uncini A, Vallat JM. Autoimmune nodo-paranodopathies of peripheral nerve: the concept is gaining ground. J Neurol Neurosurg Psychiatr 2018;89:627–35.
12. Uncini A, Santoro L. The electrophysiology of axonal neuropathies: more than just evidence of axonal loss. Clin Neurophysiol 2020;131:2367–74.
13. Van den Bergh PYK, Hadden RDM, Bouche P, et al. EFNS/PNS guideline on management of chronic inflammatory demyelinating polyradiculoneuropathy: report of a joint task force of the EFNS and the PNS - first revision. Eur J Neurol 2010; 17:356–63.
14. Tankisi H, Pugdahl K, Johnsen B, et al. Correlations of nerve conduction measures in axonal and demyelinating polyneuropathies. Clin Neurophysiol 2007; 118:2383–92.
15. Lupu VD, Mora CA, Dambrosia J, et al. Terminal latency index in neuropathy with antibodies against myelin-associated glycoproteins. Muscle Nerve 2007;35(2): 196–202.

16. EFNS/PNS guideline on management of multifocal motor neuropathy. Report of a Joint Task Force of the EFNS and the PNS - first revision. J Peripher Nerv Syst 2010;15(4):295–301.

17. Herrmann DN, Ferguson ML, Logigian EL. Conduction slowing in diabetic distal polyneuropathy. Muscle Nerve 2002;26(2):232–7.

18. Uncini A, Susuki K, Yuki N. Nodo-paranodopathy: beyond the demyelinating and axonal classification in anti-ganglioside antibody-mediated neuropathies. Clin Neurophysiol 2013;124:1928–34.

19. Sumner AJ. The physiological basis for symptoms in Guillain–Barré syndrome. Ann Neurol 1981;9(suppl):28–30.

20. Dyck PJ, Taylor BV, Davies JL, et al. Office immunotherapy in chronic inflammatory demyelinating polyneuropathy and multifocal motor neuropathy. Muscle Nerve 2015;52(4):488–97.

21. Dyck PJ, O'Brien PC, Litchy WJ, et al. Use of percentiles and normal deviates to express nerve conduction and other test abnormalities. Muscle Nerve 2001;24: 307–10.

22. Litchy WJ, Albers JW, Wolfe J, et al. Proficiency of nerve conduction using standard methods and reference values (Trial 4). Muscle Nerve 2014;50(6):900–8.

23. Model policy for needle electromyography and nerve conduction studies. Available at: https://www.aanem.org. Accessed October 12, 2020.

24. England JD, Gronseth GS, Franklin G, et al. Distal symmetric polyneuropathy: definition for clinical research. Muscle Nerve 2005;31(1):113–23.

25. Callaghan BC, Price RS, Feldman EL. Distal symmetric polyneuropathy: a review. J Am Med Assoc 2015;314:2172–81.

26. Saporta AS, Sottile SL, Miller LJ, et al. Charcot-Marie-Tooth disease subtypes and genetic testing strategies. Ann Neurol 2011;69:22–33.

27. Berciano J, Garcia A, Gallardo E, et al. Intermediate Charcot-Marie-Tooth disease: and electrophysiological reappraisal and systematic review. J Neurol 2017;264:1655–77.

28. Li J, Krajewski K, Shy ME, et al. Hereditary neuropathy with liability to pressure palsy: the electrophysiology fits the name. Neurology 2002;58:1769–73.

29. Uncini A, Kuwabara S. The electrodiagnosis of Guillain-Barré syndrome subtypes: where do we stand? Clin Neurophysiol 2018;129:2586–93.

30. Umapathi T, Lim CSJ, Ng BCJ, et al. A simplified, graded, electrodiagnostic criterion for Guillain-Barré syndrome that incorporates sensory nerve conduction studies. Sci Rep 2019;9(1):7724.

31. Kuwabara S, Sekiguchi Y, Misawa S. Electrophysiology in Fisher syndrome. Clin Neurophysiol 2017;128(1):215–9.

32. Kuwabara S, Isose S, Mori M, et al. Different electrophysiological profiles and treatment response in "typical" and "atypical" chronic inflammatory demyelinating polyneuropathy. J Neurol Neurosurg Psychiatr 2015;86(10):1054–9.

33. Allen J. The misdiagnosis of CIDP: a review. Neurol Ther 2020;9(1):43–54.

34. Mauermann ML, Sorenson EJ, Dispenzieri A, et al. Uniform demyelination and more severe axonal loss distinguish POEMS syndrome from CIDP. J Neurol Neurosurg Psychiatr 2012;83(5):480–6.

35. Olney RK, Lewis RA, Putnam TD, et al. Consensus criteria for the diagnosis of multifocal motor neuropathy. Muscle Nerve 2003;27:117–21.

36. Zivkovic SA, Ascherman D, Lacomis D. Vasculitic neuropathy-electrodiagnostic findings and association with malignancies. Acta Neurol Scand 2007;115:432–6.

Electrodiagnostic Assessment of Myopathy

Jennifer M. Martinez-Thompson, MD

KEYWORDS

- Electromyography • Electrodiagnostic testing • Myopathy
- Neuromuscular disorders • Motor unit potential • Recruitment
- Myotonic discharges • Fibrillations

KEY POINTS

- Electrodiagnostic testing serves as an extension of the neurologic examination and is guided by the clinical impression.
- This testing can be used to confirm the presence of a myopathy while excluding disease mimickers.
- Certain electrodiagnostic patterns may help narrow the differential diagnosis and direct additional testing including identifying potential targets for muscle biopsy.

 Video content accompanies this article at http://www.neurologic.theclinics.com.

INTRODUCTION

Electrodiagnostic (EDX) testing is a useful adjunct in the evaluation of suspected myopathy and serves as an extension of the neurologic examination. Although this article focuses on the EDX assessment of myopathy, having background knowledge of the clinical and laboratory features of various myopathic disorders cannot be understated. The most important components of a myopathy evaluation continue to be a comprehensive history (including family history) and the neurologic examination, which ultimately guide the EDX approach.

Myopathies are characterized by varied patterns of weakness, muscle atrophy, and additional muscular or extramuscular features depending on the underlying disorder. The most common pattern of weakness involves proximal limb muscles, affecting the ability to climb stairs, rise from a seated position, elevate the arms, or walk due to a waddling gait. There are additional patterns of weakness in myopathy that are important for the electromyographer to recognize (**Table 1**), as the presence of one of these patterns in a patient may require sampling of muscles beyond proximal limb muscles during needle electromyography (EMG). Standard initial laboratory testing in

Department of Neurology, Mayo Clinic, 200 First Street Southwest, Rochester, MN 55905, USA
E-mail address: martinezthompson.jennifer@mayo.edu

Neurol Clin 39 (2021) 1035–1049
https://doi.org/10.1016/j.ncl.2021.06.007
0733-8619/21/© 2021 Elsevier Inc. All rights reserved.

Table 1
Patterns of weakness at myopathy onset and examples/causative genes

Proximal/Limb-Girdle	Most Acquired Myopathies, Limb-Girdle Muscular Dystrophies
Distal	
Calf	Myofibrillar myopathies (DNAJB6, MYOT) Anoctaminopathy, dysferlinopathy Debrancher deficiency
Ankle dorsiflexors	Myofibrillar myopathies (CRYAB, LDB3, DES, KLHL9, MYH7) Hereditary inclusion body myopathy (GNE) Multisystem proteinopathies Myotonic dystrophy type 1 Titinopathy
Forearm/hand muscles	Myofibrillar myopathies (FLNC, TIA1) Caveolinopathy, RYR1-opathy
Scapuloperoneal	Acid maltase deficiency Central core myopathy Emery-Dreifuss dystrophy Facioscapulohumeral muscular dystrophy Limb-girdle muscular dystrophies (CAPN3, FKRP, sarcoglycans) Nemaline myopathy (some)
Distal arm/proximal leg	Inclusion body myositis
Facial/ophthalmoparesis	Congenital myopathies (centronuclear, central core) Mitochondrial myopathy Myotonic dystrophy Oculopharyngeal muscular dystrophy
Neck extensor	Isolated neck extensor myopathy Late-onset nemaline myopathy Carnitine deficiency Amyloidosis

myopathy includes a serum creatine kinase (CK), which is usually elevated with muscle fiber necrosis or increased muscle membrane permeability as seen in many acquired inflammatory or toxic myopathies, muscular dystrophies, and in some metabolic myopathies.[1]

With the increasing availability and ease of genetic testing, EDX testing and muscle biopsy may be deferred in the appropriate clinical context, such as when the suspicion for an inherited myopathy is high based on the clinical phenotype or supportive family history; this is particularly relevant in the pediatric population given the discomfort associated with these tests. However, for many patients with suspected myopathy an underlying cause cannot be established with the initial clinical evaluation and laboratory testing, highlighting the importance of EDX testing as a concurrent step in the evaluation.

EDX testing is useful in the assessment of myopathy for several reasons:

1. Confirmation of a myopathy while excluding disease mimickers (ie, motor neuron disease, motor neuropathies, and neuromuscular junction [NMJ] disorders).
2. Providing diagnostic information to narrow the differential diagnosis based on the pattern of muscle involvement and/or presence of abnormal spontaneous activity.
3. Identifying potential targets for muscle biopsy when clinical identification of weak muscles appropriate for biopsy is limited.
4. Assessing disease progression or therapy response.

In certain muscle disorders, the EDX testing may be normal (ie, corticosteroid myopathy, some mitochondrial myopathies). Having an understanding of the limitations of EDX assessment in these contexts is important in guiding subsequent assessments when appropriate.

ELECTRODIAGNOSTIC APPROACH

A stepwise approach to evaluating a patient with suspected myopathy is outlined in **Fig. 1**. In many cases, EDX testing to evaluate for myopathy is performed in conjunction with laboratory studies and other ancillary testing.

Nerve Conduction Studies

Standard nerve conduction studies

Standard NCS are commonly normal in patients with myopathy, and this includes the motor NCS, as most myopathies manifest with proximal weakness and distal muscles are the ones typically selected for study.[2] The approach to NCS in myopathy should include at least 1 motor and 1 sensory nerve in a single upper and lower limb, for example, ulnar motor (recording over abductor digiti minimi [ADM]) and median antidromic sensory and peroneal motor (recording over extensor digitorum brevis [EDB]) and sural sensory.

Low-amplitude compound muscle action potentials (CMAP) with preserved distal latencies and conduction velocities may be found in more severe and diffuse myopathies or in those that are distal predominant clinically. In critical illness myopathy (CIM) in intensive care unit (ICU) patients, diffusely low amplitude CMAPs with increased durations occur due to slowed conduction from muscle membrane inexcitability (**Fig. 2**).[3,4] Diffusely low-amplitude CMAPs in a patient with weakness can also be seen in NMJ disorders, particularly Lambert-Eaton myasthenic syndrome (LEMS). Further evaluation for an NMJ defect with repetitive nerve stimulation (RNS) studies should be pursued in that setting. Low-amplitude CMAPs are more often seen in neurogenic than myopathic process, such as motor neuron disease and motor neuropathies.[5]

Sensory NCS should be normal in an isolated myopathy. Abnormalities in these responses can be found in disorders affecting both muscle and nerve (ie, critical illness neuromyopathy) or in patients with a preexisting peripheral neuropathic process from another cause.

Repetitive nerve stimulation

When diffusely low CMAPs are present on standard motor NCS, presynaptic NMJ disorders (eg, LEMS) should be excluded with further testing. In these cases, muscles with low CMAPs are maximally exercised for 10 seconds and the corresponding motor nerves then receive a single supramaximal stimulus. If the patient is unable to follow commands, electrical stimulation at rapid rates (>20 Hz) for 10 seconds may be necessary to simulate exercise. A significant incremental response (facilitation) in the CMAP amplitude suggests a presynaptic NMJ defect. Traditionally, an increment in the CMAP amplitude greater than 100% from baseline is considered significant. Baseline 2 Hz RNS should also be performed to evaluate for decrement as would be expected in both presynaptic and postsynaptic NMJ disorders (>10% in more than 2 nerves).[6]

Some inherited myopathies also have associated neuromuscular transmission defects, including centronuclear myopathy, plectinopathy, desminopathy, *SCN4A*-myopathy, and myopathy due to certain glycosylation defects. The neuromuscular transmission defects in these patients may be partially responsive to acetylcholinesterase inhibitors or 3,4-diaminopyrimidine.[7,8] In addition, coexisting immune-mediated myopathy and acetylcholine receptor antibody–positive myasthenia gravis

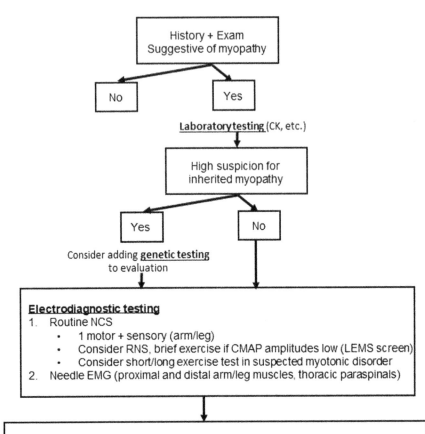

Fig. 1. Suggested approach in the clinical and electrodiagnostic evaluation of a patient with suspected myopathy.

has been more recently reported with immune checkpoint inhibitor (ICI) use in various cancer treatments.[9] Baseline and postexercise RNS of at least 2 nerves with associated muscle weakness should be performed to look for decrement in individuals with suspected ICI-associated myopathy and to consider incorporating at least baseline RNS when an inherited myopathy is suspected to identify patients that may potentially benefit from NMJ-targeted therapies.

Exercise testing

The short and long exercise tests are useful in the evaluation of patients with suspected channelopathy or nondystrophic myotonia. These exercises are traditionally

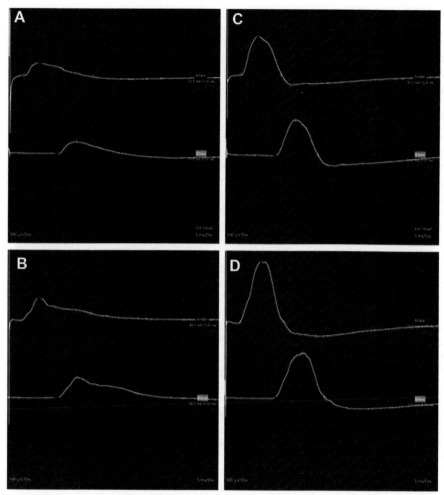

Fig. 2. Compound muscle action potentials (CMAPs) in a patient with critical illness myopathy at the time of diagnosis and after clinical improvement. (*A*) Prolonged peroneal (recording extensor digitorum brevis) CMAP duration (16 ms) and low amplitude. (*B*) Prolonged tibial (abductor hallucis) CMAP duration (19 ms). (*C, D*) Peroneal and tibial motor recordings after clinical improvement, resulting in higher amplitude and shorter duration (10 ms and 11 ms, respectively).

performed by stimulating the ulnar nerve (ADM) with several baseline trials to ensure stability of the CMAP. The short exercise test may differentiate between paramyotonia congenita and myotonia congenita. It involves the contraction of the ADM for 10 seconds followed by CMAP amplitude assessment after exercise and every subsequent 10 seconds up to 1 minute. This protocol may be repeated in suspected cases of paramyotonia congenita after cooling the limb to enhance the CMAP amplitude drop after brief exercise. The CMAP amplitude patterns after exercise vary depending on the specific channelopathy and have been previously described in detail.[10,11]

In contrast, the long exercise test is used in the assessment of individuals with periodic paralysis and is most helpful when performed in the midst of a paralytic episode. It involves contraction of the ADM for 5 minutes with several second periods of rest every

30 seconds during exercise. Serial CMAP amplitude assessment occurs immediately after exercise, every subsequent minute postexercise for 5 minutes, and then every 5 minutes for 45 minutes. In periodic paralysis, there is an initial increase in the CMAP amplitude after exercise followed by a gradual decrease in amplitude over the remainder of the study (>40% decrease from baseline).[12] With increasing use of genetic testing in the evaluation of channelopathies, exercise studies are being performed less routinely.

Needle Electromyography

The needle EMG is the most instructive portion of the EDX evaluation in myopathy, but this is contingent on mindful muscle selection guided by findings on the neurologic examination. In general, clinically weaker muscles will show the most prominent needle EMG abnormalities. Needle EMG of at least 2 proximal and 1 distal muscle in a single upper and lower limb in addition to sampling the thoracic paraspinals is recommended. The number of muscles to study depends on the pattern of weakness and in some cases will require sampling of additional muscles beyond more commonly studied muscles such as the deltoid, biceps, triceps, first dorsal interosseous, glutei, vasti, tibialis anterior, and gastrocnemius. Ideally, the serum CK should be measured before EMG, as the CK may be transiently increased if measured several hours after study completion. This increase is generally less than a 1.5-fold elevation from baseline, with return to baseline levels within 48 to 72 hours.[13]

Although the yield of needle EMG is higher when clinically weak muscles are studied, there are some situations in which the only clinically weak muscles are in sites that cannot be easily biopsied. The goal of needle EMG in those cases is to identify potential targets that are amenable to muscle biopsy based on subclinical myopathic changes or abnormal spontaneous activity.[14] Muscle selection for biopsy is mainly based on the presence of fibrillation potentials and short duration motor unit potentials (MUPs), which have been associated with histopathologic correlates of myopathy including necrotic/regenerating fibers, fiber splitting, vacuolization of muscle fibers, and inflammation.[15,16] If a muscle biopsy is performed shortly after the needle EMG, the contralateral muscle of the side studied is recommended to avoid any potential needle-related tissue artifact.[17]

The various components of the needle EMG are useful in the evaluation of a patient with suspected myopathy and include assessment of (1) insertional/spontaneous activity, (2) MUP morphology, and (3) recruitment pattern of MUPs.

Insertional/spontaneous activity

Muscle fiber irritability in various myopathic disorders can manifest as increased insertional activity, abnormal spontaneous activity, or a combination of both. The insertional activity in some myopathies may be prolonged beyond several seconds due to the instability of individual muscle fiber membranes.

Prolonged insertional activity with myotonic discharges is present most commonly in inherited myotonic disorders and in some acquired myopathies. Myotonic discharges are the action potentials of single muscle fibers and generated spontaneously with needle movement or muscle contraction. They repetitively fire at a frequency between 40 and 100 Hz over a prolonged period of time, waxing and waning in amplitude and frequency resulting in the characteristic "dive-bomber" sound (Video 1).[6]

Abnormal spontaneous activity includes positive sharp waves (PSWs) and fibrillation potentials, which in myopathy are generated from single muscle fibers after physical separation from their respective endplate zone and motor nerve terminals in the setting of necrosis, fiber splitting, or vacuolization. They can also be generated from muscle membrane irritability secondary to surrounding inflammation or necrosis.[2]

PSWs and fibrillation potentials are not specific for myopathies, as they are seen in neurogenic and some NMJ disorders. However, fibrillation potentials in myopathies may be lower in amplitude and have a slower firing rate than what is seen in neurogenic processes. In chronic myopathies, complex repetitive discharges (CRDs) may be present. These are nonspecific for myopathy, also occur in chronic neurogenic disorders, and imply the longstanding nature of the underlying process.[6]

Insertional activity may be decreased in chronic end-stage myopathy due to replacement of muscle fibers by fibrous and fatty connective tissue. End-stage muscles may be difficult to sample due to their fibrotic nature and should be avoided for muscle biopsy. Alternatively, decreased insertional activity can also occur in disorders affecting muscle membrane depolarization as seen during a periodic paralysis attack or with McArdle disease during a muscle contracture/cramp, the latter resulting in electrical silence during needle movement in the muscle.[18]

Motor unit potential morphology

In muscles affected by a myopathic process, there is either loss of muscle fibers in individual motor units or atrophy of certain muscle fiber types. In both situations the number of innervated muscle fibers within the recording region of the needle electrode is decreased, resulting in a decrease in the size of individual motor units, and this manifests as short-duration, low-amplitude MUPs. The number of phases and turns for MUPs in some myopathies may also be increased due to the asynchrony of individual muscle fiber firing from drop-out of muscle fibers or from varied conductions along the muscle membrane of individual fibers. Of the different parameters in the assessment of MUP morphology in myopathy, the MUP duration is the most important.[6]

When evaluating MUP morphology, patients are asked to activate the desired muscle at a low level of activation so that only several MUPs are recruited for analysis. Analysis of MUPs at this low level of activation is key in the assessment of myopathy, as the MUPs that are recruited later with stronger muscle contraction are generally larger in size (corresponding to type 2 muscle fibers) and may mask smaller MUPs in the background. At least 20 MUPs with an adequate rise time (0.5 ms or less) should be assessed in each muscle studied.

In chronic myopathies, intermixed normal- and long-duration MUPs with short-duration MUPs may be seen. This typically occur in more severely affected muscles, where there is enough muscle fiber loss at the motor endplates that motor nerve terminals of individual motor units attempt to reinnervate still existing muscle fibers, resulting in larger MUPs. A mixture of short-duration, low-amplitude and long-duration, and high-amplitude MUPs can also be seen in critical illness neuromyopathy, generally with neurogenic changes in a length-dependent pattern involving distal muscles and myopathic changes most prominently in proximal muscles.[19]

It is important to note that short-duration, low-amplitude MUPs are not specific for myopathies, as they can be seen in severe NMJ disorders or with nascent MUPs as part of early reinnervation after a severe neurogenic injury.

Recruitment pattern of motor unit potentials

Because individual motor units are smaller in patients with myopathy due to muscle fiber loss, the force that each motor unit can generate is decreased. To compensate for this, more motor units are activated than expected based on patient effort during attempted muscle contraction, and this results in the rapid (early) recruitment pattern seen with myopathies. Both the recruitment frequency and the firing rate of the MUPs are normal in rapid recruitment, and only the number of firing MUPs relative to the force expended is affected.[14] Rapid recruitment requires judging the patient effort.

Rarely, reduced recruitment of some MUPs may be appreciated in long-standing or severe myopathies when the extent of muscle fiber loss is so severe that only a reduced number of motor units are available to fire. Muscles showing a predominantly mixed pattern of short- and long-duration MUPs in addition to reduced recruitment should be avoided for muscle biopsy if possible, as these findings are more representative of end-stage muscle.

In some settings, quantitative EMG is used for evaluating myopathic disorders.[20] However, this technique is not used for routine clinical practice, and there are no evidence-based guidelines regarding its use. Single-fiber EMG is also not generally recommended for assessment of myopathic disorders, as abnormalities are nonspecific and could be seen in myopathic, neurogenic, or NMJ disorders.

Electromyography Patterns in Myopathies

Although individual EDX findings are nonspecific, the pattern of findings may point toward general types of myopathies; this may help narrow the differential diagnosis and allow the clinician to tailor additional diagnostic testing, including laboratory evaluation, muscle biopsy, or genetic testing.

The findings on needle EMG for various myopathic disorders can be categorized into basic patterns, although many myopathies can have overlapping patterns. These EDX patterns include the following:

1. Myopathic MUPs with fibrillation potentials
2. Myopathic MUPs without fibrillation potentials
3. Frequent myotonic discharges with or without myopathic MUPs
4. Normal EMG with clinical findings that suggest myopathy

Myopathic motor unit potentials with fibrillation potentials

Table 2 highlights various myopathies associated with frequent fibrillation potentials. The salient EDX features are summarized for several of these myopathies in the following section.

Immune-Mediated Myopathies

The immune-mediated (inflammatory) myopathies represent a heterogeneous group of acquired muscle disorders and include dermatomyositis (DM), polymyositis (PM), sporadic inclusion body myositis (sIBM), necrotizing autoimmune myopathy, and nonspecific myositis.[21] PM is a controversial entity, as it is thought to represent misdiagnosis of actual sIBM in some individuals.

These myopathies are generally characterized by prominent muscle membrane irritability, resulting in fibrillation potentials, PSWs, and occasionally myotonic discharges. The degree of spontaneous activity is thought to reflect the severity of disease activity. Short-duration, low-amplitude, polyphasic MUPs with rapid recruitment in addition to abnormal spontaneous activity are present mainly in proximal muscles for DM, PM, and nonspecific myositis, consistent with the clinical distribution of weakness. Both are treated with a combination of corticosteroids and disease modifying therapies. In treatment-responsive cases, partial improvement or resolution of fibrillation potentials may be seen.[22]

In sIBM, the quadriceps, finger flexors, and ankle dorsiflexors are involved early in the disease.[23] These muscles tend to have the most substantial changes on the needle EMG. With progression of weakness, a mixture of short-duration and long-duration MUPs may be present in a patchy fashion. Rapid recruitment is still maintained in this setting, helping to differentiate from a concomitant neurogenic process of another

Table 2
Myopathies with short-duration motor unit potentials with or without fibrillation potentials

	With Fibrillations	Without Fibrillations
Inflammatory/Immune-mediated		
Inflammatory myopathies	+	+ (treated)
Necrotizing autoimmune myopathy	+	+ (treated)
Inclusion body myositis	+	
Toxic/Endocrine		
Statins	+	
Penicillamine	+	
Chloroquine	+	
Critical illness myopathy	+	+ (milder cases)
Corticosteroid myopathy		+
Hypothyroid myopathy	+	+
Hyperthyroid myopathy		+
Infiltrative/Infectious		
Amyloid myopathy	+	+
Sarcoid myopathy	+	
Viral myositis, trichinosis	+	
Dystrophies		
Dystrophinopathies	+	
Limb-girdle muscular dystrophies	+ (some)	+ (some)
Myofibrillar myopathies	+	+
Emery Dreifuss muscular dystrophy	+	+
Facioscapulohumeral muscular dystrophy	+	+
Oculopharyngeal muscular dystrophy		+
Myotonic dystrophy type 1 and 2	+	
Congenital Myopathies		
Centronuclear myopathy	+	+
Late onset rod myopathy	+	+
Metabolic		
Acid maltase deficiency	+	+
Myophosphorylase deficiency	+	+
Carnitine deficiency	+	+
Carnitine palmitoyl transferase 2 deficiency		+
Mitochondrial myopathy	+ (some)	+ (some)

cause. Reduced recruitment of occasional short-duration MUPs may also be evident. About one-third of individuals with sIBM also have a sensorimotor axonal peripheral neuropathy as reflected on the NCS, and in this setting, more prominent neurogenic changes may be present on the needle EMG in distal lower limb muscles.

Elevated anti-5'-nucleotidase 1A (NT5C1A) antibodies have been recently described in 40% to 60% of patients with sIBM and can be a useful adjunct in diagnostic evaluation. However, as nonspecific elevation of anti-NT5C1A has been reported in other inflammatory myopathies, muscle biopsy remains the gold standard in establishing a definite diagnosis of sIBM based on the presence of rimmed vacuoles, cytoplasmic congophilic inclusions, and endomysial inflammation with autoaggressive features[23]; this makes muscle selection for biopsy important when sIBM is suspected. Muscles are ideally selected based on moderate clinical weakness, but when clinically weak muscles cannot be easily biopsied, selection of a muscle with fibrillation potentials and predominantly short duration MUPs on needle EMG is reasonable. There are no current treatments to slow the progression of sIBM.

Hereditary inclusion body myopathies (hIBM) are distinct from sIBM in pathophysiology and in clinical presentation despite pathologic and EDX similarities. Some forms of hIBM are associated with multisystem proteinopathies, which can have mixed short- and long-duration MUPs on needle EMG, given the overlapping features of hIBM and motor neuron disease in some individuals. Hereditary IBM should be considered in individuals with symptom onset earlier than age 45 years, an atypical pattern of weakness for sIBM, a serum CK greater than 10 times the upper limits of normal, or when there is a family history of weakness, amyotrophic lateral sclerosis, frontotemporal dementia, or Paget disease of the bone.[23,24]

Necrotizing Autoimmune Myopathy

Although necrotizing autoimmune myopathy (NAM) is an immune-mediated myopathy, the pathologic features on muscle biopsy of minimal inflammation and prominent muscle fiber necrosis and regeneration differentiate it from the other inflammatory myopathies. NAM presents with subacute, occasionally gradual proximal lower limb–predominant weakness and persistently elevated serum CK. Coexisting distal limb, neck flexor, and diaphragmatic weakness is common. Three serologic subtypes of NAM have been identified: anti-HMG CoA reductase (HMGCR) myopathy, antisignal recognition particle myopathy, and seronegative NAM. Anti-HMGCR myopathy can occur even in the absence of prior statin exposure. Seronegative and anti-HMGCR NAM are associated with an increased risk of cancer requiring malignancy screening.[21,22,25]

The findings on needle EMG are typically more diffuse in NAM compared with inflammatory myopathies but include fibrillation potentials and PSWs in addition to rapidly recruited short duration, low amplitude, and polyphasic MUPs. Prominent myotonic discharges may be present in some cases, particularly in anti-HMGCR myopathy. With aggressive immunosuppressive therapy, the EDX findings may improve.

NAM has also been described as a complication of ICI use in various cancer treatments, specifically with programmed cell death protein 1 (PD-1) inhibitor use and associated neuromuscular autoimmunity. The clinical and EDX features overlap with what is seen in NAM from other causes, but in some patients concurrent NMJ defects and nerve involvement are present, resulting in a confusing constellation of findings on NCS and the needle EMG. This includes abnormalities on standard NCS, decrement on RNS consistent with a postsynaptic NMJ disorder, and MUP variability on needle EMG in addition to potentially intermixed short- and long-duration MUPs in some muscles with varied recruitment patterns. Treatment with immunosuppressive therapy is necessary in conjunction with stopping the PD-1 inhibitor.[9]

Toxic or Endocrine Myopathies

Myopathies can be caused by toxicity from various drugs, some endocrine disorders, or from multifactorial factors as seen in CIM. Statins can cause asymptomatic elevation of CK but rarely may cause a direct toxic myopathy with proximal weakness or anti-HMGCR–associated NAM as described previously. The direct toxic myopathy from statins tends to improve after the agent is discontinued, whereas weakness will continually progress in NAM unless treated with immunotherapy.

Some toxic and endocrine myopathies are associated with fibrillation potentials, occasional myotonic discharges, and rapidly recruited short-duration MUPs, but most have isolated short-duration MUPs with normal spontaneous activity. Abnormal spontaneous activity has been reported in direct toxic myopathy from cholesterol-lowering agents and chloroquine/hydroxychloroquine use. In terms of endocrine disorders, hypothyroid myopathy has been associated with fibrillation potentials.[26]

CIM is an important consideration in ICU patients with generalized weakness. NCS show low-amplitude CMAPs with prolonged durations and with normal conduction velocities and distal latencies. There is sparing of the sensory NCS unless there is a concomitant peripheral neuropathy as seen in critical illness neuromyopathy (critical illness polyneuropathy). In that case, CMAP distal latency prolongation and conduction velocity slowing may be present. CIM is generally associated with fibrillation potentials but in some patients the findings are isolated to rapid recruitment of short-duration, polyphasic MUPs without fibrillation potentials.[3,4,19]

Muscular Dystrophies

Muscular dystrophies comprise inherited, progressive muscle diseases pathologically characterized by muscle fiber necrosis and gradual replacement of necrotic regions with fibrous and fatty connective tissue. For some of the dystrophies, there can be associated inflammatory changes surrounding necrotic fibers. This category of muscle disorders is broad and includes the dystrophinopathies such as Duchenne and Becker muscular dystrophy, limb girdle muscular dystrophies, myofibrillar myopathies, and facioscapulohumeral dystrophy.[27] In dystrophies with more severe phenotypes, fibrillation potentials may be present along with short-duration MUPs, but studies correlating the pattern of EDX abnormalities with specific dystrophies are lacking. In many dystrophies, fibrillation potentials may be absent and only isolated short-duration MUPs are evident. The distribution of muscles with needle EMG abnormalities may be more useful in patients with suspected muscular dystrophy than the specific abnormalities noted within muscles, highlighting the importance of sampling muscles in which clinical weakness is present.

With the advent of genetic testing, the utility of EDX testing has decreased. Although the needle EMG can confirm that there is an underlying myopathy and the distribution of changes (ie, limb girdle vs distal predominant) may suggest a general dystrophy category, it does not provide information pointing to a specific molecular defect. The limitations of EMG in this setting have become more apparent with the overlapping dystrophy and congenital myopathy phenotypes reported with various genetic abnormalities.[28,29]

Congenital and Metabolic Myopathies

Of the congenital myopathies, the centronuclear and late-onset rod myopathies most commonly have fibrillation potentials in addition to rapidly recruited short-duration MUPs. Of the various lipid and glycogen storage disorders, carnitine, acid maltase, and myophosphorylase deficiency (McArdle disease) may have fibrillation potentials.[2]

Myopathic motor unit potentials without fibrillation potentials

Table 2 highlights various myopathies without associated fibrillation potentials. Many of these overlap with what is seen in the first pattern. Most congenital, mitochondrial, endocrine, and toxic myopathies have isolated short-duration MUPs without fibrillation potentials. The lack of fibrillation potentials suggests the indolent nature of the underlying process. In addition, partially treated or fully treated inflammatory or necrotizing myopathies may have this pattern.

Frequent myotonic discharges with or without myopathic motor unit potentials
Box 1 highlights various muscle disorders associated with frequent myotonic discharges. The salient EDX features are summarized for several of these disorders in the following section.

Dystrophic and Nondystrophic Myotonias

Myotonic disorders include the myotonic dystrophies (DM1 and DM2), which are multisystem disorders exhibiting progressive fixed muscle weakness, atrophy, and clinical myotonia. Most patients with DM1 and DM2 have electrical myotonia, although this may be sparse in individuals with DM2. In DM1, the electrical myotonia may be so prominent that it is difficult to evaluate the morphology of underlying MUPs. Although the electrical myotonia can be diffuse, it is present mainly in distal limb muscles for DM1 and in proximal leg muscles for DM2. The classic waxing-waning myotonic discharges are common in DM1, whereas in DM2 waning discharges have been more frequently described. Short-duration, low-amplitude, polyphasic MUPs with rapid recruitment are generally present in affected muscles.[30,31]

The nondystrophic myotonias (muscle channelopathies) are due to mutations in various ion channels and include myotonia congenita, paramyotonia congenita, and potassium-aggravated myotonias; these can manifest with muscle stiffness, myotonia, or episodic weakness due to various dietary, temperature, or activity-related triggers. Diffuse electrical myotonia may be identified in these conditions and may become more prominent along with fibrillation potentials after limb cooling in myotonia congenita and paramyotonia congenita. The MUPs may be normal or short in duration. The short and long exercise tests are useful in differentiating between the nondystrophic myotonias and may direct genetic testing, although with the expansion of genetic testing panels the exercise tests are used less frequently to assist with diagnosis.[32]

Muscle channelopathies also include the periodic paralyses, which are characterized by flaccid paralysis or focal weakness lasting for minutes to hours triggered by certain dietary intake, activity, temperature, or emotional states. Clinical and electrical myotonia may be present in hyperkalemic periodic paralysis at the onset or in between paralysis attacks, but myotonic is absent in hypokalemic periodic paralysis. Unless there is static weakness in the setting of repeated and severe attacks, the MUP morphology on needle EMG is typically normal. The long exercise test is most useful in the assessment of suspected periodic paralysis.[12,32]

Box 1
Muscle disorders with frequent myotonic discharges on electromyography

With Clinical Myotonia
  Myotonic dystrophy type 1 and 2
  Myotonia congenita
  Paramyotonia congenita

Without Clinical Myotonia
  Hyperkalemic periodic paralysis
  Acid maltase deficiency
  Potassium sensitive myotonia
  Toxic myopathies (eg, statins, fibrates, colchicine, hydroxychloroquine, penicillamine)
  Inflammatory/necrotizing myopathies
  Centronuclear myopathy
  Caveolinopathy

Acid Maltase Deficiency

Acid maltase deficiency (acid alpha-glucosidase deficiency or Pompe disease) results in a metabolic myopathy presenting with severe weakness early in life or later in childhood or adulthood. CK levels in adult-onset acid maltase deficiency may be normal, and the proximal-predominant pattern of weakness may make it difficult to distinguish from other myopathies. A clinical clue is early respiratory muscle involvement, resulting in dyspnea on exertion or orthopnea. Axial weakness may also be present. Because recombinant enzyme treatment exists for these patients, screening patients with myopathy for acid alpha-glucosidase deficiency by evaluating the acid alpha-glucosidase activity with simple dried blood spot testing is often recommended.

Needle EMG in acid maltase deficiency may show abnormal spontaneous activity ranging from fibrillation potentials to myotonic discharges and CRDs in proximal muscles for early onset cases. In contrast, myotonic discharges and fibrillations may be limited to the paraspinal muscles in adult-onset cases or in those with a milder phenotype.[33]

Normal electromyography with clinical findings that suggest myopathy

Table 3 highlights various myopathies in which EDX testing may be normal. These myopathies are generally not associated with muscle fiber necrosis or inflammation and span metabolic, endocrine, congenital, and mitochondrial causes.[34,35] Corticosteroid myopathy is most commonly associated with a normal EMG despite clinical evidence of proximal weakness, whereas in some cases short-duration MUPs are present in proximal muscles. The normal EMG findings are thought to be due to the isolated type 2 fiber atrophy that occurs with corticosteroid use.[36] The analysis of MUPs in myopathy is mainly limited to type 1 fibers, as type 1 fibers are the first to be recruited with muscle contraction. Because MUPs generated from type 1 fibers are already present when type 2 fibers are subsequently recruited, the former will conceal any potential type 2 fiber-related abnormalities.

Table 3
Myopathies with normal electromyography

Type of Myopathy	Examples
Type 2 muscle fiber atrophy	Corticosteroid myopathy, disuse atrophy
Mitochondrial myopathies (some)	-
Congenital myopathies (some)	-
Metabolic myopathies	Myophosphorylase deficiency, carnitine palmitoyl transferase 2 deficiency

SUMMARY

EDX evaluation is a useful adjunct in the evaluation of patients with suspected myopathy. The main roles of EDX testing are to confirm the presence of a myopathy while excluding disease mimickers and to help narrow the differential diagnosis based on the EDX pattern; this helps to target subsequent laboratory evaluation and genetic testing and to identify potential muscle biopsy targets in the appropriate clinical context. It also provides a baseline for subsequent assessment of disease progression or response to therapy.

CLINICS CARE POINTS

- An initial neurologic examination in a patient with suspected myopathy is a must in guiding the approach to EDX testing including specific muscle selection for needle EMG.

- Include assessment of both spontaneous activity and voluntary muscle on needle EMG in all muscles tested.
- EDX abnormalities beyond short duration MUPs may be present in myopathic disorders and should be factored into the clinical context.

DISCLOSURE

Dr J.M. Martinez-Thompson has no conflicts of interests to disclose.

SUPPLEMENTARY DATA

Supplementary data to this article can be found online at https://doi.org/10.1016/j.ncl.2021.06.007.

REFERENCES

1. Barohn RJ, Dimachkie MM, Jackson CE. A pattern recognition approach to the patient with a suspected myopathy. Neurol Clin 2014;32(3):569–vii.
2. Lacomis D. Electrodiagnostic approach to the patient with suspected myopathy. Neurol Clin 2012;30:641–60.
3. Goodman BP, Harper CM, Boon AJ. Prolonged compound muscle action potentials duration in critical illness myopathy. Muscle Nerve 2009;40:1040–2.
4. Lacomis D. Electrophysiology of neuromuscular disorders in critical illness. Muscle Nerve 2013;47:452–63.
5. Daube JR, Rubin DI. Electrodiagnosis of Muscle Disorders. In: Engel AG, Franzini-Armstrong C, editors. Myology. Third edition. New York: McGraw Hill; 2004.
6. Rubin DI. Assessing the motor unit with needle electromyography. In: Daube JR, Rubin DI, editors. Clinical neurophysiology. Third Edition. New York: Oxford University Press; 2009. p. 403–50.
7. Nicolau S, Kao JC, Liewluck T. Trouble at the junction: when myopathy and myasthenia overlap. Muscle Nerve 2019;60:648–57.
8. Elahi B, Laughlin RS, Litchy WJ, et al. Neuromuscular transmission defects in myopathies: rare but worth searching for. Muscle Nerve 2019;59:475–8.
9. Kao JC, Brickshawana A, Liewluck T. Neuromuscular complications of programmed cell death-1 (PD-1) inhibitors. Curr Neurol Neurosci 2018;18:63.
10. Fournier E, Arzel M, Sternberg D, et al. Electromyography guides toward subgroups of mutations in muscle channelopathies. Ann Neurol 2004;56(5):650–61.
11. Fournier E, Viala K, Gervais H, et al. Cold extends electromyography distinction between ion channel mutations causing myotonia. Ann Neurol 2006;60(3):356–65.
12. McManis PG, Lambert EH, Daube JR. The exercise test in periodic paralysis. Muscle Nerve 1986;9(8):704–10.
13. Levin R, Pascuzzi RM, Bruns DE, et al. The time course of creatine kinase elevation following concentric needle EMG. Muscle Nerve 1987;10:242–5.
14. Paganoni S, Amato A. Electrodiagnostic evaluations of myopathies. Phys Med Rehabil Clin N Am 2013;24:193–207.
15. Sener U, Martinez-Thompson J, Laughlin RS, et al. Needle electromyography and histopathologic correlation in myopathies. Muscle Nerve 2019;59:315–20.
16. Naddaf E, Milone M, Mauermann ML, et al. Muscle biopsy and electromyography correlation. Front Neurol 2018;9:839.

17. Engel WK. Focal myopathic changes produced by electromyographic and hypodermic needles. Arch Neurol 1967;16:509–11.

18. Rowland LP, Araki S, Carmel P. Contracture in McArdle's disease: Stability of adenosine triphosphate during contracture in phosphorylase-deficient human muscle. Arch Neurol 1965;13(5):541–4.

19. Kramer CL, Boon AJ, Harper CM, et al. Compound muscle action potential duration in critical illness neuromyopathy. Muscle Nerve 2018;57:395–400.

20. Nandedkar SD, Stalberg EV, Sanders D. Quantitative EMG. In: Dumitru D, Amato AA, Swartz MJ, editors. Electrodiagnostic medicine. 2nd edition. Philadelphia: Hanley & Belfus; 2002. p. 293–356.

21. Milone M. Diagnosis and management of immune-mediated myopathies. Mayo Clin Proc 2017;92:826–37.

22. Pinal-Fernandez I, Casal-Dominguez M, Mammen AL. Immune-mediated necrotizing myopathy. Curr Rheum Rep 2018;20:21.

23. Weihl CC. Sporadic inclusion body myositis and other rimmed vacuolar myopathies. Continuum 2019;25:1586–98.

24. Nicolau S, Liewluck T. TFG: at the crossroads of motor neuron disease and myopathy. Muscle Nerve 2019;60:645–7.

25. Kassardjian CD, Lennon VA, Alfugham NB, et al. Clinical features and treatment outcomes of necrotizing autoimmune myopathy. JAMA Neurol 2015;72:996–1003.

26. Katzberg HD, Kassardjian CD. Toxic and endocrine myopathies. Continuum 2016;22:1815–28.

27. Butterfield RJ. Congenital muscular dystrophy and congenital myopathy. Continuum 2019;25(6):1640–61.

28. Liewluck T, Milone M. Untangling the complexity of limb-girdle muscular dystrophies. Muscle Nerve 2018;58:167–77.

29. Milone M, Liewluck T. The unfolding spectrum of inherited distal myopathies. Muscle Nerve 2019;59:283–94.

30. Logigian EL, Ciafaloni E, Quinn LC, et al. Severity, type, and distribution of myotonic discharges are different in type 1 and type 2 myotonic dystrophy. Muscle Nerve 2007;35:479–85.

31. Young NP, Daube JR, Sorenson EJ, et al. Absent, unrecognized, and minimal myotonic discharges in myotonic dystrophy type 2. Muscle Nerve 2010;41:758–62.

32. Heatwole CR, Statland JM, Logigian EL. The diagnosis and treatment of myotonic disorders. Muscle Nerve 2013;47:632–48.

33. Kassardjian CD, Engel AG, Sorenson EJ. Electromyographic findings in 37 patients with adult-onset acid maltase deficiency. Muscle Nerve 2015;51:759–61.

34. Cohen BH. Mitochondrial and metabolic myopathies. Continuum 2019;25:1732–66.

35. Milone M, Wong LJ. Diagnosis of mitochondrial myopathies. Mol Genet Metab 2013;110:35–41.

36. Gupta A, Gupta Y. Glucocorticoid-induced myopathy: Pathophysiology, diagnosis and treatment. Indian J Endocrinol Metab 2013;17:913–6.

Electrodiagnostic Assessment of Neuromuscular Junction Disorders

Hans D. Katzberg, MD, MSc, FRCPC[a],*, Alon Abraham, MD[b]

KEYWORDS

- Neuromuscular junction • Myasthenia gravis • Single-fiber electromyography
- Repetitive nerve stimulation • SFEMG • RNS

KEY POINTS

- Repetitive nerve stimulation is a commonly available test with adequate specificity for postsynaptic and presynaptic neuromuscular junction transmission defects.
- Single-fiber electromyography can accurately identify disorders of neuromuscular junction transmission, such as myasthenia gravis, Lambert-Eaton myasthenic syndrome and botulism.
- Novel methods of neuromuscular junction testing are being investigated and include ocular vestibular myogenic potentials and electrooculography.

INTRODUCTION

Electrophysiology plays a critical role in the assessment of disorders of the neuromuscular junction (NMJ), including myasthenia gravis (MG) and Lambert-Eaton myasthenic syndrome (LEMS) (**Table 1**).[1] In the 1940s, Harvey and Masland[2] used repetitive nerve stimulation (RNS) to assess neuromuscular disorders, including MG, and, although these techniques have been refined, the basic tenets remain unchanged. In the 1960s, Stalberg and Eskedt[3] developed single-fiber electromyography (SFEMG), a technique that assesses the integrity of the NMJ by recording the variation in interpotential intervals (IPIs) between adjacent single muscle fiber action potentials.[4] Modifications to SFEMG methodology have included the use of disposable concentric needles to estimate jitter and stimulated SFEMG, which is useful in patients who are not able to cooperate with voluntary contraction.

Genetic testing and antibody testing for myasthenic disorders have improved greatly over time; however, electrophysiology remains the sole or first-line diagnostic

---

[a] Division of Neurology, University Health Network, Toronto General Hospital, 200 Elizabeth Street, 5ES-306, Toronto, Ontario M5G 2C4, Canada; [b] Neuromuscular Diseases Unit, Department of Neurology, Tel Aviv Sourasky Medical Center, 6 Weizmann Street, Tel Aviv 6423906, Israel
* Corresponding author.
E-mail address: hans.katzberg@utoronto.ca

Neurol Clin 39 (2021) 1051–1070
https://doi.org/10.1016/j.ncl.2021.06.013
0733-8619/21/© 2021 Elsevier Inc. All rights reserved.

Table 1
Disorders of the neuromuscular junction

Medical Conditions	Toxic/Medications
MG	Botulinum toxin (iatrogenic)
• Generalized	Hypermagnesemia
• Ocular	
LEMS	Organophosphate poisoning
Botulism	Snake envenomation
• Foodborne	
• Wound	
Congenital myasthenic syndromes	Acetylcholinesterase inhibitor overdose

test in many clinical settings (**Box 1**). This article reviews RNS and SFEMG and introduces other developing methods for the assessment of NMJ dysfunction, including ocular vestibular myogenic evoked potentials (oVEMPs)[5] and oculography.[6] In-depth details relating to RNS and SFEMG are discussed in seminal monographs,[7,8] textbooks,[1,9] and guidelines.[10,11]

REPETITIVE NERVE STIMULATION
Rationale and Pathophysiology

Muscle activation requires adequate release of acetylcholine (ACh) molecules from the presynaptic nerve terminal, diffusion across the synaptic cleft, and binding to ACh receptors on the postsynaptic muscle membrane to produce a sufficient endplate potential (EPP).[1] The safety factor is the EPP amplitude above the threshold required to generate a muscle fiber action potential; this is reduced in postsynaptic NMJ disorders, such as MG (**Fig. 1**).[12] Low-frequency (<5-Hz) RNS, results in a decrement in EPPs with repetitive stimuli (**Fig. 2**). In presynaptic disorders, EPPs may be low at baseline, and increased by brief, high-intensity exercise or rapid (30–50 Hz) RNS by mobilizing more Ach from secondary stores. Thus, the technique of RNS can help to assess NMJ integrity and identify a presynaptic or postsynaptic disorder.

Technical Aspects

When performing RNS, limb temperature should be maintained above 33°C, because cold temperature may decrease acetylcholinesterase enzyme function and reduce test sensitivity. Anticholinesterase medications should be withheld 12 hours prior to

Box 1
Situations assessed initially with electrodiagnostic testing

- MG or LEMS, where antibody testing is not readily available or delayed
- Ocular MG (often antibody negative)
- Seronegative MG or LEMS
- Congenital myasthenic syndromes (when genetic testing is negative or not available)
- Toxic NMJ transmission disorders
- Foodborne or wound botulism, prior to confirmatory assay or assay not available

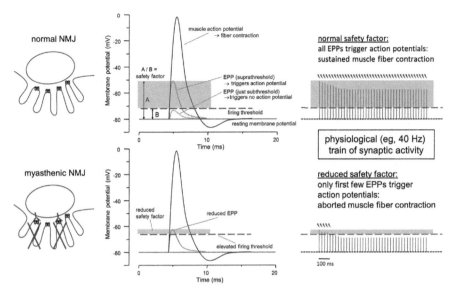

Fig. 1. Electrophysiologic function of a healthy NMJ (*top*) and a myasthenic NMJ (*bottom*). The large safety factor in normal NMJs results in elicitation of all muscle fiber action potentials (red flashes [*right panels*]), even with a decrease in EPP amplitude, during high stimulation rates. In the myasthenic NMJ, smaller EPPs and elevated firing threshold reduce the safety factor, resulting in transmission failure with rapid simulation. (*From* Plomp JJ. Trans-synaptic homeostasis at the myasthenic neuromuscular junction. Front Biosci (Landmark Ed) 2017;22:1033-1051; with permission.)

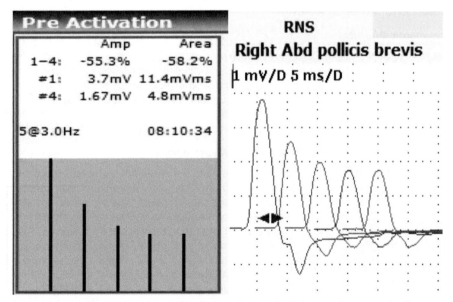

Fig. 2. Decrement of 55.3% in amplitude (Amp) and 58.2% in area between the first and fourth responses with low-frequency (3-Hz) stimulation of the median nerve, recording from the right abductor (Abd) pollicis brevis in a patient with MG. D, division.

testing, if possible.[10] Movement of the limb, stimulator, or recording electrodes during stimulation can result in inconsistent compound muscle action potential (CMAP) recordings. Limb immobilization can be performed by securing the limb to a board or with a strap and securing the electrodes with tape.[9] Supramaximal nerve stimulation should be ensured, and the muscle should be at rest during stimulation. Any recorded decrement should be reproducible to ensure reliability.[8]

Repetitive Nerve Stimulation Nerve/Muscle Selection

Although any motor nerve can be used for RNS, those used most commonly are the ulnar, median, musculocutaneous, axillary, spinal accessory, and facial nerves.[9] The optimal muscle chosen is a symptomatic, weak muscle.[13] Examining proximal or facial muscles and multiple muscles increases test sensitivity.[14] Several studies have shown superior sensitivity for facial RNS in ocular MG, in contrast to proximal limb muscles in generalized MG,[14–16] although these findings are not uniform.[17] Test sensitivity also is affected by disease severity and is lower in patients with very mild or pure ocular symptoms. In these cases, SFEMG may be considered as the initial test to diagnose NMJ impairment.[10]

Postsynaptic Disorders

Standard RNS techniques for assessing postsynaptic NMJ disorders include slow RNS (<5 Hz) with trains of 5 and up to 10 stimuli.[9] Although short (10 seconds) of exercise may result in transient, immediate improvement in baseline decrement, more prolonged exercise (30 seconds–1 minute), repeating RNS trains every minute for 3 minutes to 5 minutes, may produce increased decrement, which gradually improves back to the baseline decrement value (**Fig. 3**). Studies have shown that activation can increase RNS sensitivity by 7% to 15%[13,18,19]; however, drawbacks to repeated postactivation stimulations include additional time and discomfort. Testing additional nerve-muscle combination at baseline if the first is normal also has been shown to increase sensitivity by up to 15%.[19]

Presynaptic Disorders

Decrement on slow RNS also is common in presynaptic disorders, such as LEMS.[20,21] The electrophysiologic hallmark of LEMS is low baseline CMAP amplitudes and post-exercise facilitation, which can be demonstrated after 10 seconds of maximum voluntary contraction (**Fig. 4**). In patients who are unable to exercise a muscle adequately or in situations where additional confirmation of presynaptic dysfunction is required, 30-Hz to 50-Hz stimulation may be required in order to demonstrate facilitation (see **Fig. 4**).

Abnormal Repetitive Nerve Stimulation in Myasthenia Gravis

In normal subjects, slow RNS results in consistent generation of motor unit action potentials owing to a large safety factor, and no CMAP amplitude/area decrement should be present. Therefore, any reproducible decrement in should raise a suspicion of NMJ dysfunction.[9] Studies have shown that in normal subjects, amplitude decrement may reach up to 2%, whereas area decrement may reach up to 6%[22]; therefore, RNS amplitude measurement might be preferred to area measurement. Characteristic decrement is U-shaped, because there is stabilization or even improvement in decrement after the fifth or sixth stimulus (**Fig. 5A**). Sudden or irregular variations between consecutive responses should raise suspicion of a technical artifact (see **Fig. 5B**).

To avoid false-positive test results, a cutoff value of greater than 10% has been recommended to confirm NMJ impairment.[10] The sensitivity of RNS for diagnosing NMJ impairment using this 10% traditional cutoff is higher in generalized MG (53%–89%)

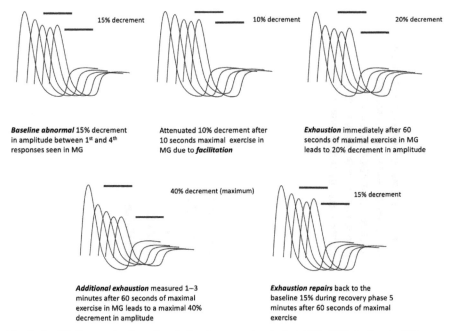

Baseline abnormal 15% decrement in amplitude between 1st and 4th responses seen in MG

Attenuated 10% decrement after 10 seconds maximal exercise in MG due to **facilitation**

Exhaustion immediately after 60 seconds of maximal exercise in MG leads to 20% decrement in amplitude

Additional exhaustion measured 1–3 minutes after 60 seconds of maximal exercise in MG leads to a maximal 40% decrement in amplitude

Exhaustion repairs back to the baseline 15% during recovery phase 5 minutes after 60 seconds of maximal exercise

Fig. 3. Facilitation and exhaustion following exercise during 3-Hz RNS studies in MG.

versus ocular MG (20%–67%).[23] Studies have shown that a lower cutoff value of greater than 7% can increase sensitivity from 7% to 20% while maintaining a specificity of greater than 90%,[17,24] with some investigators considering a lower cutoff value of greater than 5%.[25] Based on these data, it appears that considering lower cutoffs of 5% to 10% could be considered to confirm NMJ impairment if technical factors and clinical context are considered carefully.

Abnormalities in Other Neuromuscular Junction Disorders

Abnormal postexercise facilitation is suggestive of presynaptic dysfunction in LEMS. Using a threshold of 100% increment in baseline CMAP amplitude with short duration (10 seconds), exercise can help distinguish pathologic from physiologic

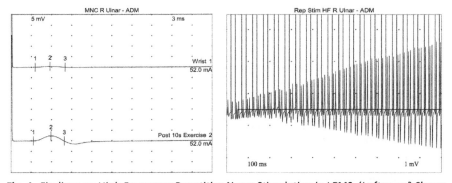

Fig. 4. Findings on High Frequency Repetitive Nerve Stimulation in LEMS. (*Left panel*) Shows an ulnar motor amplitude increment of 200% after 10 seconds of exercise. (*Right panel*) Shows an amplitude increase of 950% with 50-Hz RNS. ADM, adductor digiti minimi.

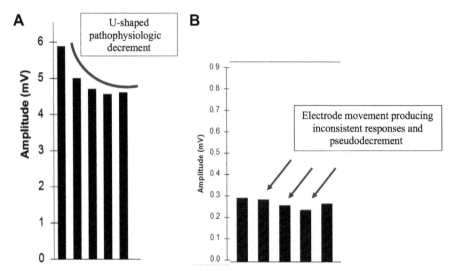

Fig. 5. (*A*) Physiologic decrement with largest amplitude decrement between first and second responses and less prominent decrement subsequently until the 4th response and slight improvement by the fifth response, generating a U-shaped appearance. (*B*) Inconsistent stimulator or recording electrode movement producing nonphysiologic pseudodecrement.

pseudofacilitation, which can reach up to 30% of baseline CMAP.[10] Some studies have shown that a lower cutoff of 60% increment may increase sensitivity from 85% to 97% while maintaining a high specificity of 99%. Similar cutoff values apply to 30-Hz to 50-Hz stimulation; however, brief maximum voluntary contraction is preferred in cooperative patients due to the pain associated with high-frequency stimulation.[26] Similar increment findings can be seen in botulism,[27] and presynaptic congenital disorders of the NMJ (CMS),[28] as can the decremental responses seen with slow-frequency RNS. In congenital slow-channel syndrome and congenital acetylcholinesterase deficiency, prolongation of the end plate potential (EPP) may produce a repetitive CMAP after single stimulation because the EPP duration exceeds the refractory period of the action potential (**Fig. 6**).

SINGLE-FIBER ELECTROMYOGRAPHY
Rationale and Pathophysiology

The development of a multielectrode single-fiber needle allowed for recording of adjacent single-fiber action potentials over a recording surface of approximately 300 μm.[3] The smaller recording area of SFEMG needles compared with the smallest concentric needles allows for individual muscle fiber pair comparison (**Fig. 7**). By using this needle as well as signal trigger and delay techniques, the variation in time for pairs of EPPs to reach threshold can be measured, termed *neuromuscular jitter*. Jitter is measured as the mean consecutive difference (MCD) of IPIs (**Fig. 8**).[3] Although there is an intrinsic physiologic jitter for each muscle (**Fig. 9**), a disruption in neuromuscular transmission leads to abnormally elevated jitter (**Fig. 10**).[29] When neuromuscular transmission is impaired to the point that the EPP is not sufficient to generate an action potential along a fiber, blocking of a fiber occurs, which results in muscle weakness (**Fig. 11**).

Technical Aspects

SFEMG uses a high-pass filter of 500 Hz to eliminate low-frequency components from distal muscle fibers and allow more selective recording of muscle fiber pairs.[7]

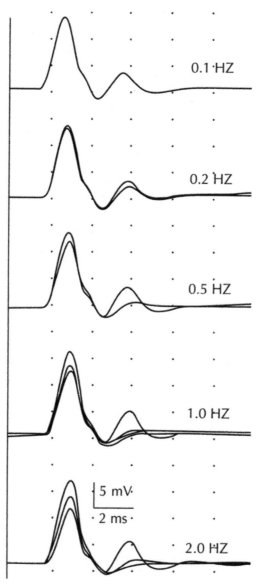

Fig. 6. Repetitive discharges in the abductor digiti quinti muscle in a patient with congenital acetylcholinesterase deficiency. Four consecutive superimposed CMAPs are shown with increasing stimulus rates. Stimulation faster than 0.5 Hz abolishes the repetitive discharge. (*From* Engel AG. Myasthenia gravis and myasthenic disorders. In: Harper CM, editor. Electrodiagnosis of myasthenic disorders. New York: Oxford University Press; 2012. p. 37–59; with permission.)

Potentials should meet certain criteria to accurately obtain jitter (**Table 2**),[8] and a minimum of 50 (ideally 100) consecutive voluntarily activated consecutive potentials is recommended for an accurate estimate of jitter and blocking. Twenty individual jitter recordings per muscle are recommended to determine if a muscle has NMJ defect,

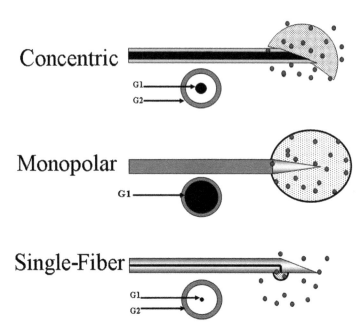

Fig. 7. Single-fiber, concentric, and monopolar needle electrodes and recording areas. G1 denotes recording electrode and G2 reference electrode. (*From* Rubin DI. Needle electromyography: basic concepts and patterns of abnormalities. Neurol Clin. 2012;30(2):429-456. https://doi.org/10.1016/j.ncl.2011.12.009; with permission.)

which usually requires 2 to 4 needle insertions. Jitter values of each pair can be displayed in tables or histograms (**Fig. 12**). Studies have shown that 15 pairs may be sufficient to determine if a test is normal[30]; however, attention should be placed on assuring appropriate fiber pairs are collected because technical factors can lead to falsely elevated jitter. Pitfalls and errors in measuring jitter are reviewed by Stålberg and colleagues[31] and are summarized in **Table 3**.

Abnormal versus Normal Single-fiber electromyography

Age-adjusted normal jitter values for commonly tested muscles used in SFEMG have been published (**Table 4**).[32,33] An SFEMG test is considered abnormal if any of the

$$MCD = \frac{(IPI_1 - IPI_2) + (IPI_2 - IPI_3) + \ldots\ldots\ldots (IPI_{n-1} - IPI_n)}{n - 1}$$

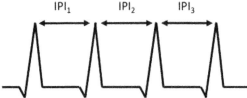

Fig. 8. MCD calculation based on IPI of consecutively firing single-fiber action fiber potentials.

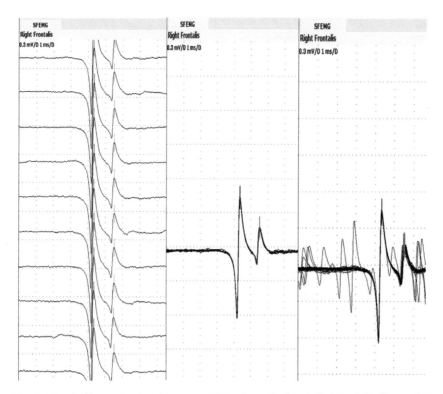

Fig. 9. Muscle fiber pairs showing normal jitter from the frontalis (26 μs). (*Left panel*) Shows 10 individual and middle panel shows 10 superimposed fiber pairs from the recording. (*Right panel*) shows the 100 superimposed pairs used to calculate jitter. D, division.

following criteria is met: (1) more than 10% of pairs (eg, at least 3 out of 20 pairs) exceed the upper limit of normal, (2) mean jitter is increased compared with control mean jitter values for the same muscle, or (3) any pairs with blocking are observed.

Specificity of Single-fiber electromyography

Abnormal SFEMG is nonspecific and also can be seen in neuropathic or myopathic conditions[34,35] (**Box 2**). This makes it critical to consider the clinical presentation and findings on routine electrophysiological tests (NCS and needle electromyography [EMG]) when interpreting SFEMG. Abnormal SFEMG cannot distinguish between pre-synaptic and postsynaptic NMJ disorders.

Sensitivity of Single-fiber Electromyography in Generalized Myasthenia Gravis

Despite limited specificity, the sensitivity of SFEMG is high for MG. This is true w particularly hen testing clinically weak muscles where a normal SFEMG test can be helpful to exclude neuromuscular transmission defect related to MG. Even if clinically unaffected, the extensor digitorum communis has a sensitivity between 78% and 90%.[7,36] Because many patients with GMG have ocular weakness, selection of 1 or more facial muscles (eg, frontalis or orbicularis oculi) as a primary or secondary site is appropriate.[37,38] Rarely, SFEMG of multiple facial muscles are normal in GMG,[7] highlighting the need to consider additional extremity muscles if

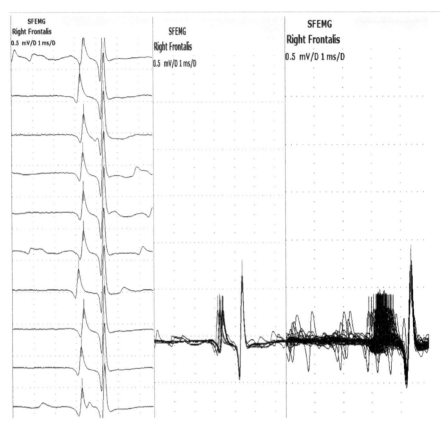

Fig. 10. Ten individual (*left panel*) and superimposed (*middle panel*) muscle fiber pairs showing increased jitter without blocking in the frontalis during SFEMG. (*Right panel*) Shows 100 superimposed pairs with mean jitter of 85 μs. D, division.

the clinical suspicion of MG is high. SFEMG can be normal with mild or transient MG symptoms, prompting the importance of repeat testing if symptoms persist or progress.[8]

Sensitivity of Single-fiber Electromyography in Ocular Myasthenia Gravis

SFEMG of the facial muscle ocular MG shows sensitivities ranging from 90% to 100%,[39,40] with sensitivities of 93% for mild, 96% for moderate, and 100% for severe ocular dysfunction in a series 117 patients with ocular MG.[40]

Longitudinal Single-fiber Electromyography and Correlation with Myasthenia Gravis Severity

Studies that have demonstrated a relationship between SFEMG jitter and clinical outcomes in MG[7] as well as a response to MG-specific treatments.[41] The painful nature of the test, occasional discrepancy between clinical features and jitter, and advances in clinical outcome measure development for MG make serial SFEMG for assessment of MG status rare outside the research setting. Early studies determined that a fall in jitter of 10% was associated with clinical improvement in MG,[7] and a recent study set the

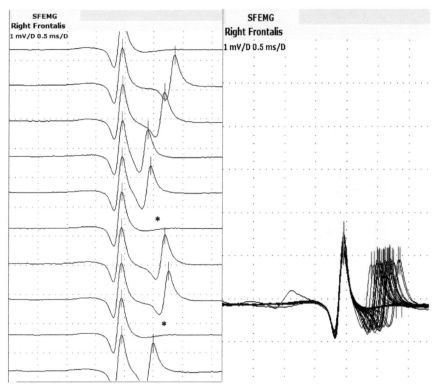

Fig. 11. Ten superimposed (*left panel*) and individual (*right panel*) muscle fiber pairs showing increased jitter and blocking (*) in the frontalis during voluntary contraction.

Table 2
Criteria for adequate selection of action potentials for inclusion in conventional, concentric-needle, and stimulated single-fiber electromyography assessment of jitter

General Single-fiber Electromyography Requirements	Concentric-needle Single-fiber Electromyography Requirements	Stimulated Single-fiber Electromyography Requirements
• Amplitude >200 μV • Rise time <300 μs • Single-fiber action potentials <4 ms from triggered potential • Collect 15–20 pairs	• Individual spikes should have positive and negative peaks • Constant slope of initial rising phase, without notches • Well-defined signal peaks with constant shape • No visible amplitude variation on consecutive discharges • Constant baseline preceding and following signal to avoid risk that signal is affected by other activated motor units	• When an abnormal pair is identified, maintain stimulus intensity above the liminal value • Increase stimulation intensity until the jitter value no longer changes • Adjustment of stimulus strength to avoid coactivation of nearby axons • Collect 30 minimum jitter values obtained with positional changes of stimulating and recording electrodes • Stimulation frequency, 10 Hz

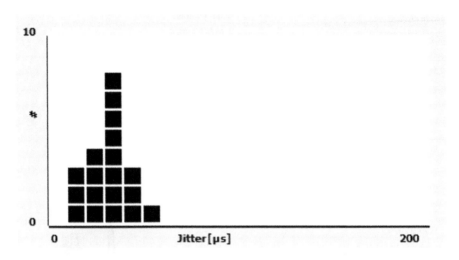

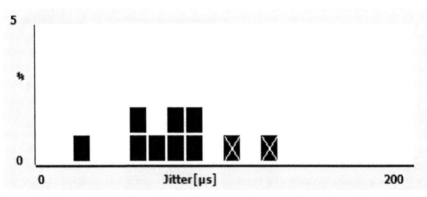

Fig. 12. (*Top*) Normally distributed jitter histogram of muscle fiber pairs collected from the frontalis, mean jitter 32 μs. (*Bottom*) Abnormally distributed jitter histogram from 10 muscle fiber pairs demonstrating 60% abnormal pairs, 20% blocking pairs (boxes with X) and elevated mean jitter of 91 μs.

minimum clinical important difference for clinical improvement at a jitter value from the frontalis at 14.2 μs, or 16% change from the mean.[42]

Single-fiber Electromyography in Non–Myasthenia Gravis Junction Disorders

Abnormal SFEMG commonly is seen in LEMS and can be helpful in arriving at the diagnosis.[26] In LEMS, high pretreatment mean jitter and the proportion of abnormal or blocked pairs correlate with CMAP amplitude and increment on 50-Hz RNS.[7] SFEMG plays a major diagnostic role in cases of suspected botulism toxicity given the potential for severe or fatal outcomes if not identified or treated in a timely fashion. In these cases, SFEMG shows disrupted NMJ transmission in nearly all cases even early in the diagnosis when bioassays still may be under investigation.[27] Electrophysiology also is key in the early identification of CMS, where genetic testing is limited or not available.[43] In these cases, SFEMG can be helpful to detect NMJ defect but is not

Table 3
Pitfalls in single-fiber electromyography jitter measurement in conventional single-fiber electromyography, concentric-needle single-fiber electromyography, and stimulated single-fiber electromyography

General pitfalls	
Superimposition of many spikes	Essential to record jitter from well separated individual spikes. Summation of 2 or more spikes causes error in jitter measurement, more likely seen in CN-SFEMG due to larger recording area
Positive waves	Positive triangular waves following single-fiber action potentials have increased jitter and blocking and should not be included for analysis because they are components of the immediately preceding spike.
Ongoing reinnervation	Immature axonal branches and endplates undergoing reinnervation have increased jitter and should not be included, particularly in distal muscles, which are more prone to denervation.
Riding signals	If a second signal spike begins during the falling phase of the first, this is known as a riding potential, where the amplitude level trigger occurs at different times leading to falsely elevated jitter.
Recordings with low jitter	Jitter values <5 μs sometimes can be related to branches of a longitudinally split muscle fiber on voluntary SFEMG and direct stimulation with stimulated SFEMG.
Voluntary activation pitfalls	
Influence from the triggering spike	When recording voluntary signals from 3 or more spikes, increased jitter in the triggering spike can cause falsely elevated mean jitter. Thus, normal jitter from voluntary signals with 3 or more spikes can be accepted, but if abnormal these should be discounted.
Velocity recovery function effect	With higher interdischarge intervals, a phase of increased velocity (velocity recovery function) increases jitter falsely with irregular firing rates. In this situation, the mean sorted difference, calculated along with the MCD, is more accurate. Due to velocity recovery function, jitter values >150 μs should be set to 150 μs and IPI should be <4 ms when calculating the mean jitter.
Dual IPI latency, the flip-flop phenomenon	Bimodal latency of the IPI can lead to short latency jumps in healthy subjects and long latency jumps in the setting of reinnervation and falsely elevated jitter.

(continued on next page)

Table 3 *(continued)*	
Electrical stimulation pitfalls	
Insufficient stimulation	If electrical stimulus intensity is weak, impulse initiation is uncertain and falsely increased jitter and pseudoblocking can occur. This can be minimized by increasing the stimulus intensity minimally.
Velocity recovery function effect	Although the constant firing rate with stimulated SFEMG eliminates velocity recovery function effects, a change in the rate shortens the latency of spikes during the first second after rate change and should not be counted.
Axon reflex	In normal or pathologic settings, the evoked spike can occur at variable latency positions due to an axon reflex and lead to falsely elevated jitter.

Data from Stålberg E, Sanders DB and Kouyoumdjian JA. Pitfalls and errors in measuring jitter. Clinical Neurophysiology 2017 128:2233-41.

be able to distinguish between the presynaptic and postsynaptic CMS, which requires RNS.

Concentric-needle Single-fiber Electromyography

The high cost and theoretic risk of infection with SFEMG needles has prompted investigation into the use of disposable concentric-needle electrodes for assessment of NMJ dysfunction.[7] By using the concentric needles with smallest recording area and applying filters in the 1 K-Hz to 10 K-Hz range, concentric-needle SFEMG (CN-SFEMG) can be used as an accurate estimate of jitter. CN-SFEMG has supplanted

Table 4 Age-adjusted reference values for jitter measurements in healthy subjects during voluntary muscle activation (microseconds): 95% CI for upper limit of mean consecutive difference/95% CI for mean consecutive difference values of individual fiber pairs									
Age (years)	10 y	20 y	30 y	40 y	50 y	60 y	70 y	80 y	90 y
Frontalis	33.6/49.7	33.9/50.1	34.4/51.3	35.5/53.5	37.3/57.5	40.0/63.9	43.8/74.1		
Orbicularis oculi	39.8/54.6	39.8/54.7	40.0/54.7	40.4/54.8	40.9/55.0	41.8/55.3	43.0/55.8		
Extensor digitorum communis	34.9/50.0	34.9/50.1	35.1/50.5	35.4/51.3	35.9/52.5	36.6/54.4	37.7/57.2	39.1/61.1	40.9/66.5

Adapted from AAEM Quality Assurance Committee. American Association of Electrodiagnostic Medicine. Literature review of the usefulness of repetitive nerve stimulation and single fiber EMG in the electrodiagnostic evaluation of patients with suspected myasthenia gravis or Lambert-Eaton myasthenic syndrome. Muscle Nerve 2001;24(9):1239-47; with permission.

Box 2
Non-neuromuscular junction disorders with abnormal single-fiber electromyography

- Peripheral neuropathies (during reinnervation)
- Motor neuron disease (especially amyotrophic lateral sclerosis during periods of early reinnervation)
- Hereditary myopathies, in particular dystrophic processes
- Metabolic myopathies (jitter can be increased during attacks of weakness)
- Focal or diffuse myositis

---

conventional SFEMG in many centers as a diagnostic NMJ assessment tool.[44–46] Recently, normal controls for commonly tested muscles have been collected among a group of 20-year-old to 80 year-old healthy participants (**Table 5**).[47] Criteria for acceptable CN-SFEMG signals are listed in **Table 2**, and common pitfalls and artifacts encountered when selecting CN-SFEMG signals are listed in **Table 3**. Positive predictive value of abnormal CN-SFEMG has been shown to be 0.93 with negative predictive value of 0.76, indicating that abnormal CN-SFEMG is useful in confirming MG; however, it may be more limited in excluding MG if normal. Given the superior sensitivity of facial over limb CN-SFEMG for GMG, facial muscles are recommended as the primary and secondary muscles tested when using this modality.

Simulated Single-fiber Electromyography

Voluntary SFEMG requires sustained, low-intensity contraction of the muscle being studied, which is challenging in cooperative adults and nearly impossible in children, patients who are unconscious, patients who are not able to cooperate with the test, or those with impairments, such as tremor. In these situations, stimulated SFEMG can be considered, which involves stimulating a terminal motor branch using surface or monopolar needle electrodes and measuring jitter in a distally supplied muscle using an SFEMG needle. In order to recruit and measure reliable, supramaximal muscle pairs, stimulations of 2 Hz to 10 Hz are applied, and intensity adjusted to collect a minimum of 30 pairs. Normal values for stimulated conventional and CN-SFEMG[47,48] have been established in commonly tested muscles, including orbicularis oculi, frontalis

---

Table 5
Summary of upper limits of normal for stimulated and voluntary concentric-needle electrode single-fiber electromyography

Muscle Tested	Oribularis Oculi	Frontalis	Extensor Digitorum Communis
Voluntary			
Mean MCD (μs)	31	28	30
Eighteenth MCD (μs)	45	38	43
Stimulated			
Mean MCD (μs)	27	21	24
Twenty-seventh MCD (μs)	36	28	35

Adapted from Stålberg E, Sanders DB, Ali S, et al. Reference values for jitter recorded by concentric needle electrodes in healthy controls: A multicenter study. Muscle Nerve 2016;53(3):351-62; with permission.

and extensor digitorum (see **Table 5**), as have criteria for adequate execution of the test (see **Table 2**) and pitfalls (see **Table 3**).

Stimulated Potential Analysis with Concentric-needle Electrodes

A variation of stimulated SFEMG is stimulated potential analysis with concentric-needle electrodes (SPACE), which uses monopolar motor nerve stimulation with low stimulation potential of less than 1 mA and a frequency of 10 Hz.[49] MCD then can be calculated from multiple muscle fiber pairs simultaneously, minimizing the needle insertions, saving time, and obviating cooperation. Due to these advantages, the technique is useful particularly in children, where this technique increasingly has been used. The most commonly studied paradigm is stimulation of the facial nerve and recording from the orbicularis oculi, which also confers advantage because the stimulation and recording sites are behind a child's visual field of view.

Practical Single-fiber Electromyography Considerations

Medications can affect SFEMG. Pyridostigmine can lead to false-negative results in mild MG and should be held for at least 12 hours prior to the study.[8] Botulinum toxin,

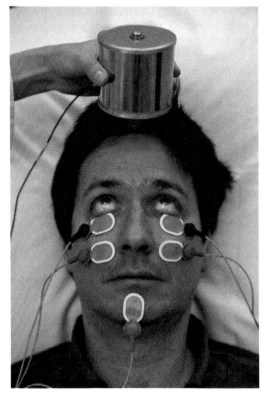

Fig. 13. Experimental setup for oVEMPs. Recording is performed in sustained upgaze as in the Simpson test, thus activating the superior rectus and inferior oblique muscles in both eyes. A minishaker at the hairline of the forehead delivers the bone-conducted vibration stimulus. Active (black) and reference (red) electrodes measure the surface EMG signal from the inferior oblique muscles; ground electrode (green) is on the chin. (*From* Valko Y, Rosengren SM, Jung HH, et al. Ocular vestibular evoked myogenic potentials as a test for myasthenia gravis. Neurology 2016; 86:660–8; with permission.)

used for treatment of headache, wrinkles, dystonia, or spasticity, can lead to iatrogen-ically increased jitter.[50] Although this usually transiently disrupts only the muscles injected, there are data showing disruption of NMJ transmission in muscles distant to those injected and remote to the time of treatment.[51] Devices, such as deep brain stimulators, can interfere with recording, particularly of facial muscles, and should temporarily be switched off during testing if safe to do so.[52]

NOVEL METHODS TO ASSESS NEUROMUSCULAR JUNCTION TRANSMISSION
Ocular Vestibular Evoked Myogenic Potentials

oVEMPs traditionally have been used to test otolith function. By applying 4-milli-second (ms) bursts of 500-Hz bone-conducted skull vibration delivered by a handheld minishaker positioned over the hairline, ocular myogenic potentials can be recorded from active electrodes over the infraorbital margins (**Fig. 13**).[5] Using 10-stimuli recording at 20 Hz, oVEMP signals have shown decrement in patients with a small group of patients with MG compared with controls.

Oculography

Electrooculography signals use the cornea-retina as an electric dipole and is used in the assessment of various neurologic conditions where ocular movement is affected. Electrooculography analysis has been shown to measure abnormal characteristics of extraocular muscle action potentials and response to edrophonium in patients with MG.[6,53]

SUMMARY

RNS and SFEMG continue to be useful tests, which help confirm and evaluate NMJ disorders, such as MG and LEMS. RNS has lower sensitivity than SFEMG but is more helpful in distinguishing between presynaptic and postsynaptic NMJ defects. Although SFEMG is the most sensitive test, specificity is limited, and the test cannot distinguish between presynaptic and postsynaptic disorders. Novel methods, including Ocular vestibular-evoked myogenic potential (oVEMP) analysis and oculog-raphy assessments, currently are under investigation and have potential future value in the assessment of NMJ diseases.

CLINICS CARE POINTS

- RNS has the best sensitivity when testing weak muscles or testing more than 1 muscle.

- Conventional SFEMG and CN-SFEMG are more sensitive but less specific than RNS for assessment of NMJ disorders and cannot distinguish reliably between presynaptic and postsynaptic conditions.

- If SFEMG is not possible due to inability to cooperate with adequate voluntary activation, stimulated SFEMG can be considered.

DISCLOSURE

The authors have nothing to disclose.

REFERENCES

1. Stålberg E. Clinical neurophysiology of disorders of muscle and neuromuscular junction, including fatigue. Amsterdam: Elsevier; 2004.

2. Harvey AM, Masland RL. A method for the study of neuromuscular transmission in human subjects. Bull Johns Hopkins Hosp 1941;68:81–93.

3. Ekstedt J. Human single muscle fiber action potential. Acta Physiol Scand 1964; 61(suppl):226, 1–96.

4. Ekstedt J, Nilsson G, Stålberg E. Calculation of the electromyographic jitter. J Neurol Neurosurg Psychiatry 1974;37:526–39.

5. Valko Y, Rosengren SM, Jung HH, et al. Ocular vestibular evoked myogenic potentials as a test for myasthenia gravis. Neurology 2016;86:660–8.

6. Barton JJ. Quantitative ocular tests for myasthenia gravis: a comparative review withdetection theory analysis. J Neurol Sci 1999;155:104–14.

7. Sanders DB, Howard JF. AAEE minimonograph #25: single-fiber electromyography in myasthenia gravis. Muscle Nerve 1986;9:809–19.

8. Sanders DB, Arimura K, Cui L, et al. Guidelines for single fiber EMG. Clin Neurophysiol 2019;130(8):1417–39.

9. Preston DC. RNS and SFEMG. In: Electromyography and neuromuscular disorders: clinical-electrophysiologic correlations. 3rd edition. Place: Publisher; 2012. p. 529–40.

10. Chiou-Tan FY, Tim RW, Gilchrist JM, et al. Practice parameter for repetitive nerve stimulation and single fiber EMG evaluation of adults with suspected myasthenia gravis or Lambert-Eaton myasthenic syndrome: Summary statement. Muscle Nerve 2001;24(9):1236–8.

11. AAEM Quality Assurance Committee. American Association of Electrodiagnostic Medicine. Literature review of the usefulness of repetitive nerve stimulation and single fiber EMG in the electrodiagnostic evaluation of patients with suspected myasthenia gravis or Lambert-Eaton myasthenic syndrome. Muscle Nerve 2001;24(9):1239–47.

12. Plomp JJ. Trans-synaptic homeostasis at the myasthenic neuromuscular junction. Front Biosci (Landmark Ed 2017;22:1033–51.

13. Oh SJ, Nagai T, Kizilay F, et al. One-minute exercise is best for evaluation of post-exercise exhaustion in myasthenia gravis. Muscle Nerve 2014;50(3):413–6.

14. Bou Ali H, Salort-Campana E, Grapperon AM, et al. New strategy for improving the diagnostic sensitivity of repetitive nerve stimulation in myasthenia gravis. Muscle Nerve 2017;55(4):532–8.

15. Misra UK, Kalita J, Srivastava A. A study of diagnostic yield, technical ease and patient discomfort of low rate repetitive nerve stimulation test in patients with myasthenia gravis. Electromyogr Clin Neurophysiol 2006;46(6):337–41.

16. Costa J, Evangelista T, Conceição I, et al. Repetitive nerve stimulation in myasthenia gravis–relative sensitivity of different muscles. Clin Neurophysiol 2004; 115(12):2776–82.

17. Lamb CJ, Rubin DI. Sensitivity and Specificity of Repetitive Nerve Stimulation with Lower Cutoffs for Abnormal Decrement in Myasthenia Gravis. Muscle Nerve 2020;62(3):381–5.

18. Rubin DI, Hentschel K. Is exercise necessary with repetitive nerve stimulation in evaluating patients with suspected myasthenia gravis? Muscle Nerve 2007;35(1): 103–6.

19. Abraham A, Alabdali M, Alsulaiman A, et al. Repetitive facial nerve stimulation in myasthenia gravis 1 min after muscle activation is inferior to testing a second muscle at rest. Clin Neurophysiol 2016;127(10):3294–7.

20. Tim RW, Massey JM, Sanders DB. Lambert-Eaton myasthenic syndrome: Electrodiagnostic findings and response to treatment. Neurology 2000;54(11):2176–8.

21. Oh SJ, Hatanaka Y, Ito E, et al. Post-exercise exhaustion in Lambert-Eaton myasthenic syndrome. Clin Neurophysiol 2014;125(2):411–4.

22. Baumann F, Henderson RD, Tremayne F, et al. Effects of prolonged repetitive stimulation of median, ulnar and peroneal nerves. Muscle Nerve 2010;41(6): 785–93.

23. Stålberg E, van Dijk H, Falck B, et al. Standards for quantification of EMG and neurography. Clin Neurophysiol 2019;130(9):1688–729.

24. Abraham A, Alabdali M, Alsulaiman A, et al. Repetitive nerve stimulation cutoff values for the diagnosis of myasthenia gravis. Muscle Nerve 2017;55(2):166–70.

25. Amandusson Å, Elf K, Grindlund ME, et al. Diagnostic Utility of Repetitive Nerve Stimulation in a Large Cohort of Patients with Myasthenia Gravis. J Clin Neurophysiol 2017;34(5):400–7.

26. Oh SJ, Kurokawa K, Claussen GC, et al. Electrophysiological diagnostic criteria of Lambert-Eaton myasthenic syndrome. Muscle Nerve 2005;32(4):515–20.

27. Padua L, Aprile I, Monaco ML, et al. Neurophysiological assessment in the diagnosis of botulism: usefulness of single-fiber EMG. Muscle Nerve 1999;22(10): 1388–92.

28. Kosac A, Gavillet E, Whittaker RG. Neurophysiological testing in congenital myasthenic syndromes: A systematic review of published normal data. Muscle Nerve 2013;48(5):711–5.

29. Sanders DB. Clinical neurophysiology of disorders of the neuromuscular junction. J Clin Neurophysiol 1993;10:167–80.

30. Abraham A, Breiner A, Barnett C, et al. Recording Fewer Than 20 Potential Pairs with SFEMG May Suffice for the Diagnosis of Myasthenia Gravis. J Clin Neurophysiol 2017;34(5):408–12.

31. Stålberg E, Sanders DB, Kouyoumdjian JA. Pitfalls and errors in measuring jitter. Clin Neurophysiol 2017;128:2233–41.

32. Gilchrist J, Barkhaus PE, Bril V, et al. Single fiber EMG reference values: a collaborative effort. Muscle Nerve 1992;15:151–61.

33. Bromberg MB, Scott DM. Single fiber EMG reference values: reformatted in tabular form. AD HOC Committee of the AAEM Single Fiber Special Interest Group. Muscle Nerve 1994;17(7):820–1.

34. Mercelis R. Abnormal single-fiber electromyography in patients not having myasthenia: risk for diagnostic confusion? Ann N Y Acad Sci 2003;998:509–11.

35. Ukachoke C, Ashby P, Basinski A, et al. Usefulness of single fiber EMG for distinguishing neuromuscular from other causes of ocular muscle weakness. Can J Neurol Sci 1994;21(2):125–8.

36. Murga L, Sánchez F, Menéndez C, et al. Diagnostic yield of stimulation and voluntary single-fiber electromyography in myasthenia gravis. Muscle Nerve 1998; 21(8):1081–3.

37. Padua L, Caliandro P, Di Iasi G, et al. Reliability of SFEMG in diagnosing myasthenia gravis: Sensitivity and specificity calculated on 100 prospective cases. Clin Neurophysiol 2014;125:1270–3.

38. Oh SJ, Kim DE, Kuruoglu R, et al. Diagnostic sensitivity of the laboratory tests in myasthenia gravis. Muscle Nerve 1992;15:720–4.

39. Hiroko K, Hatanaka Y, Sonoo M, et al. Comparison between frontalis and orbicularis oculi regarding sensitivity of voluntary single-fiber EMG for the diagnosis of ocular myasthenia gravis. Muscle Nerve 2007;36:593–4.

40. Katzberg HD, Bril V. A comparison of electrodiagnostic tests in ocular myasthenia gravis. J Clin Neuromuscul Dis 2005;6(3):109–13.

41. Juel VC, Sanders DB, Hobson-Webb LD, et al. Marked clinical and jitter improvement after eculizumab in refractory myasthenia. Muscle Nerve 2017;56:E16–8.
42. Katzberg H, Barnett C, Merkiers SJ, et al. Minimal clinically important difference in myasthenia gravis: outcomes from a randomized trial. Muscle Nerve 2014; 49(5):661–5.
43. Caldas VM, Heise CO, Kouyoumdjian JA, et al. Electrophysiological study of neuromuscular junction in congenital myasthenic syndromes, congenital myopathies, and chronic progressive external ophthalmoplegia. Neuromuscul Disord 2020;30(11):897–903.
44. Stålberg E, Sanders DB. Jitter recordings with concentric needle electrodes. Muscle Nerve 2009;40:331–9.
45. Benatar M, Hammad M, Doss-Riney H. Concentric-needle single-fiber electromyography for the diagnosis of myasthenia gravis. Muscle Nerve 2006;34:163–8.
46. Guan Y, Ding Q, Liu M, et al. Single-fiber EMG with concentric electrodes in lambert-eaton myasthenia. Muscle Nerve 2017;56(2):253–7.
47. Stålberg E, Sanders DB, Ali S, et al. Reference values for jitter recorded by concentric needle electrodes in healthy controls: A multicenter study. Muscle Nerve 2016;53(3):351–62.
48. Valls-Canals J, Povedano M, Montero J, et al. Stimulated single-fiber EMG of the frontalis and orbicularis oculi muscles in ocular myasthenia gravis. Muscle Nerve 2003;28(4):501–3.
49. Pitt M. Neurophysiological Assessment of Abnormalities of the Neuromuscular Junction in Children. Int J Mol Sci 2018;19(2):624.
50. Ruet A, Durand MC, Denys P, et al. Single-fiber electromyography analysis of botulinum toxin diffusion in patients with fatigue and pseudobotulism. Arch Phys Med Rehabil 2015;96(6):1103–9.
51. Lange DJ, Rubin M, Greene PE, et al. Distant effects of locally injected botulinum toxin: a double-blind study of single fiber EMG changes. Muscle Nerve 1991; 14(7):672–5.
52. Sadeghian H, Chitnis S, Elliott JL. Deep brain stimulation artifact in needle electromyography. Arch Neurol 2010;67(8):1030.
53. Liang T, Boulos MI, Murray BJ, et al. Analysis of electrooculography signals for the detection of Myasthenia Gravis. Clin Neurophysiol 2019;130(11):2105–13.

Electrodiagnostic Assessment of Motor Neuron Disease

Xuan Kang, MD, Dianna Quan, MD*

KEYWORDS

- Motor neuron disease • Amyotrophic lateral sclerosis • Nerve conduction studies
- Electromyography • Motor unit number estimate • Neurophysiologic index

KEY POINTS

- Electrodiagnostic testing helps to distinguish motor neuron diseases from other disorders and provides guidance for treatment.
- In patients with amyotrophic lateral sclerosis, abnormalities may be seen on motor nerve conduction studies, repetitive nerve stimulation, needle electromyography and single fiber electromyography, as well as motor unit number estimate and neurophysiologic index.
- Specific features on electrodiagnostic studies are associated with different types of motor neuron diseases.

INTRODUCTION

Motor neuron diseases (MND) are a heterogeneous group of disorders affecting the voluntary motor system, including frontal cortex motor neurons, anterior horn cells, cranial motor nerve nuclei, and corticospinal and corticobulbar tracts. The distribution of motor system injury varies depending on the specific disorder.[1,2] MND may be hereditary or acquired. Amyotrophic lateral sclerosis (ALS), the most common MND in adults, can be either sporadic or inherited and involves both upper motor neurons (UMN) and lower motor neurons (LMN). Spinal muscular atrophy (SMA), a hereditary cause of LMN degeneration, is the most common MND in children.[1–3] Other examples of hereditary diseases with diffuse motor neuron degeneration include spinal bulbar muscular atrophy, Friedreich ataxia, spinal cerebellar ataxia, multisystem atrophy, and hereditary spastic paraparesis.[1,3] In addition, infection with enterovirus species (poliovirus, coxsackie A and B, EV-D68 and A71), West Nile virus, herpes viruses, and Creutzfeldt–Jakob syndrome, are known to cause motor neuron damage.[1,4–6] Cervical spondylosis, syringomyelia, tumor, infarct, congenital dysplasia of the spinal cord, and Hirayama disease are all known to cause focal motor neuron

Department of Neurology, University of Colorado Denver, Academic Office 1, 12631 East 17th Avenue, Mailstop B185, Aurora, CO 80045, USA
* Corresponding author.
E-mail address: dianna.quan@cuanschutz.edu

Neurol Clin 39 (2021) 1071–1081
https://doi.org/10.1016/j.ncl.2021.06.008
0733-8619/21/© 2021 Elsevier Inc. All rights reserved.

dysfunction.[1,2,4] Other conditions, such as multifocal motor neuropathy with conduction block, can mimic the clinical and examination features of LMN disease.

These disorders carry very different prognoses and accurate diagnosis is crucial for appropriate management. Physical findings point to pathology in different parts of the motor system. UMN dysfunction results in hyperactive reflexes, increased tone, and weakness with preserved muscle bulk. In contrast, LMN degeneration results in flaccid weakness and fasciculations with muscle atrophy owing to a direct loss of muscle innervation. The tempo of disease onset and systemic symptoms such as fever or delirium are helpful for distinguishing acute infectious syndromes from more slowly progressive degenerative disorders. Associated findings, such as prominent sensory disturbances, cognitive changes, or bowel or bladder dysfunction, may further aid classification. Family history may provide information about possible hereditary disorders, although the absence of similar problems in family members does not preclude a genetic basis for the disease. The diagnostic strategy for MND depends on the history and examination features in individual patients. Evaluation may involve targeted imaging of the nervous system, blood work, spinal fluid analysis, genetic testing, or other modalities, but electrodiagnostic (EDX) testing is central for making an early, accurate diagnosis.

The motor unit, defined as the anatomic element consisting of an anterior horn cell, its axons and branches, the neuromuscular junctions, and all the muscle fiber innervated by the axon is the primary focus of clinical EDX testing in MND.[7] Routine clinical methods of assessing the motor unit include nerve conduction studies (NCS), needle electromyography (EMG), and repetitive nerve stimulation (RNS). Other EDX assessment tools used primarily in clinical and basic research settings include motor unit number estimate (MUNE), the neurophysiologic index (NI), and electrical impedance myography (EIM). This review focuses on the EDX assessment of ALS and selected acquired and hereditary motor neuron syndromes.

AMYOTROPHIC LATERAL SCLEROSIS

ALS is the most common MND, with approximate prevalence of 2 in 100,000 and average symptom onset around the seventh decade.[8] The disease normally starts in 1 body region, usually in a single limb, with complaints of difficulty performing daily functions and LMN or UMN findings on examination. Over subsequent months to years, symptoms spread contiguously to other limbs, bulbar, and respiratory muscles with mean survival of 2 to 4 years from symptom onset.[4] Although UMN symptoms and signs are a prerequisite for diagnosis and contribute significantly to morbidity, the LMN loss is the main contributor to rapid progressive weakness and disability.[9–11] As motor neurons die, compensatory reinnervation of abandoned muscle fibers by adjacent surviving neurons occurs via collateral sprouting. If disease progression is relatively slow, compensatory reinnervation may keep pace with neuronal loss for a time. In this case, motor neuron dysfunction may be evident on EDX testing long before clinical weakness is seen. For this reason, the most widely used ALS criteria, including the Revised El Escorial Criteria and Awaji Criteria for ALS, incorporate EDX findings in the diagnostic matrix.[12,13] The detailed discussion of ALS in this article illustrates many central concepts in the electrodiagnosis of all motor neuron disorders.

Nerve Conduction Study

An NCS is an essential component of the EDX evaluation in ALS and helps to exclude alterative diagnoses such as multifocal motor neuropathy with conduction block. On motor NCS, the compound motor action potential (CMAP) amplitude reflects combined effects of denervation, muscle atrophy, and reinnervation. The CMAP amplitude starts to decrease when reinnervation is unable to keep pace with ongoing muscle denervation and correlates with muscle strength, as well as functional disability in patients with ALS.[1,2,10,11,14] However, as the amplitude and area of the CMAP reflects the volume of innervated muscle fibers, it is insensitive for detecting early compensated motor neuron loss.

A slowed proximal conduction time may be observed in patients with ALS owing to secondary demyelinating changes close to the motor neuron.[11,15] Prolonged F-wave latency and decreased persistence have also been reported in MND.[11,16] When severe motor fiber loss drastically decreases CMAP amplitudes, phase cancellation and proximal slowing may cause amplitude differences between proximal and distal stimulation sites. Using CMAP area measurements is more useful in these cases, because area is less affected by dispersion.[2] In general, a conduction velocity less than 70% of the lower normal limits or proximal conduction block are not features associated with ALS and are more suggestive of treatable demyelinating neuropathy.[17]

In patients with ALS, prolonged distal motor latency is shown to be negatively correlated with strength and is observed even in muscles without clinical weakness. Intramuscular regeneration of thin motor axons with slowed conduction may explain this finding.[11,18] No particularly increased susceptibility to nerve compression is thought to occur in ALS.[19] One peculiarity seen in patients with ALS is the "split hand pattern," or preferential wasting of the thenar muscles with relative sparing of hypothenar muscles. As a result, significantly lower CMAP amplitudes may be observed recording the abductor pollicis brevis compared with the abductor digiti minimi muscle, with a decrease in the CMAP amplitude ratio of abductor pollicis brevis:abductor digiti minimi.[20] The split hand may also be observed in other diseases with anterior horn cell degeneration, such as SMA and spinal cerebellar ataxia, and may result from an intrinsic vulnerability of spinal motor neurons supplying the thenar complex.[21]

Even though ALS primarily results in motor neuron degeneration, minor abnormalities of sensory NCS are relatively common. In 30% to 40% of patients with ALS, sural SNAP amplitude and conduction velocity may be decreased.[22,23] In a retrospective series of 103 patients with ALS, one-third had clinical sensory symptoms or findings.[23] Of 22 patients who underwent sural nerve biopsy, 91% had abnormalities, mostly axonal degeneration and regeneration with secondary mild segmental demyelination.[23] The longitudinal study does not suggest progressive worsening, especially relative to a decrease in motor function.[16] Although these findings suggest that mild clinical or EDX sensory abnormalities may be seen in ALS, more significant sensory EDX abnormalities require an alternate explanation.

Electromyography

Evaluation by needle EMG is crucial in patients with ALS. The presence of spontaneous activity at rest is an important feature; fibrillation potentials, positive sharp waves, fasciculation potentials (FPs), complex repetitive discharges, and occasionally myotonia may all be seen in ALS. Fibrillation potentials and positive sharp waves are frequently seen. Neither type of potential is specific to ALS, but both are common in settings of active axonal and neuronal injury or muscle fiber degeneration. Early in ALS, fibrillation potentials may be sparse owing to adequate reinnervation by collateral sprouting. Careful search for such potentials may require extra time and patience.[1,2]

FPs are an important feature in ALS. These potentials represent sporadic electrical activity from activation of individual LMNs. Although FPs can be seen with many other disorders, they are sometimes the earliest EDX finding in ALS and may occur before other motor unit potential (MUP) changes.[24,25] Anterior horn cells are the origin of FPs early in ALS, but nerve terminals may also be a source later.[2] The FPs of ALS are typically unstable, long duration, and polyphasic in morphology; accompanying fibrillation and positive sharp wave potentials are common.[2] In the initial stages of disease, FP frequency remains relatively constant despite a progressive decrease in the number of viable motor neurons. In some cases, continued formation of unstable axonal sprouts may result in more abundant FPs as limb weakness progresses.[26] With further muscle atrophy, FPs eventually wane and may disappear.

Other forms of spontaneous activity observed in ALS include complex repetitive discharges and very occasionally myotonia. Spontaneous, time-locked, regularly repeating complex repetitive discharges potentials are associated with chronic muscle or nerve diseases and, when present in ALS, are observed in patients with a longer disease duration. Myotonic discharges may be seen rarely and are mostly brief in ALS, often associated with or resembling fibrillation potentials.[1,2]

During voluntary muscle activation, the characteristic EMG finding in ALS is decreased motor unit recruitment, defined as a reduction in the available number of motor units available to generate a muscle contraction. In healthy individuals, the rate of individual MUP firing increases with increased muscle force generation, followed by the orderly recruitment of additional motor units. As progressive motor neuron loss occurs in ALS, fewer motor units are available to be recruited. Muscle force generation increasingly relies on recruitment of the fewer remaining motor units firing at faster rates. This process gives rise to an important hallmark of neurogenic disease, higher recruitment ratios, defined as the firing rate of the fastest firing motor unit divided by the number of distinct motor units observed on the EMG screen.[1,2,16] After most motor neurons have degenerated, a needle EMG may demonstrate single motor unit firing rates as high as 50 Hz.[2]

As motor neurons degenerate and recruitment decreases, there is a concomitant alteration of the MUP morphology. Continued motor neuron degeneration triggers compensatory collateral spouting by the remaining neurons with the formation of immature nerve terminals. Compared with other neurogenic diseases, reinnervation in ALS is less effective owing to metabolic abnormalities at the level of anterior horn cells.[16] These newly formed terminals have a slowed conduction velocity and intermittent blocking of neuromuscular transmission, resulting in asynchronous firing of muscle fibers with polyphasic and unstable MUPs on EMG.[2,24] Increased mean motor unit duration reflects this muscle fiber asynchrony and is one way of detecting early reinnervation in ALS.[25] As more collateral sprouts develop and mature, each motor unit begins to encompass larger and larger volumes of muscle; the resulting MUPs become larger, longer, and less polyphasic as muscle fibers fire in greater synchrony.[2] The MUP recruitment and morphologic changes described are common to other neurogenic disorders besides ALS, but the combination of widespread spontaneous activity with decreased recruitment of unstable MUPs in the same distribution reflects the classic ongoing degeneration and reinnervation seen in ALS.

Repetitive Nerve Stimulation and Single Fiber Electromyography

RNS and single-fiber EMG, important in the diagnosis of neuromuscular junction disorders, are usually unnecessary in the clinical evaluation of ALS. However, abnormalities on RNS and single-fiber EMG shed light on the pathophysiology of ALS. Decremental CMAP response to slow (2–3 Hz) RNS is known to occur in ALS.[16,27,28] This abnormality is attributed to a reduced safety factor of neuromuscular transmission in the setting of newly formed axonal sprouts at immature neuromuscular junctions. Some studies suggest that more than one-half of patients with ALS may have decrement on RNS and that decremental response is as commonly seen in ALS as in myasthenia gravis.[27,28] Similar to the CMAP amplitude differences in different hand muscles, a 2-Hz RNS decrement is most strikingly observed in the abductor pollicis brevis, to a lesser degree in the first dorsal interosseous muscle, and least in the abductor digiti minimi.[29,30] The percent decrement in the CMAP area is generally greater than the CMAP amplitude, and the degree of decrement correlates with decline in strength.[30] The RNS decrement is not specific to ALS and also is seen in other motor neuron disorders such as spinal bulbar muscular atrophy and SMA, reflecting pathophysiologic changes in terminal motor axon and motor endplate function.[30–32] By contrast, nerve injury from cervical spine disease, which may have NCS and clinical examination findings similar to ALS, is not associated with significant decremental response on a 2-Hz RNS.[33] The underlying processes resulting in abnormal RNS in ALS are also measurable on single-fiber EMG, where increased jitter and blocking are observed. This sign can be an early demonstration of active reinnervation in patients with ALS.[25] Predictably, increased jitter is less prominent in cervical spine disease compared with ALS.[34]

Specialized Testing

The EDX techniques described elsewhere in this article are available in most academic centers and many community-based practices and are extremely useful for diagnosis of ALS and other MNDs; they are less helpful for monitoring disease progression or evaluating the effects of specific treatments. Additional specialized electrophysiologic techniques have been developed to further improve testing sensitivity, although these modalities have not been widely adopted in clinical practice and are primarily used only at specialized ALS treatment and research centers.

Neurophysiologic index

The NI reflects denervation and reinnervation secondary to axonal degeneration. It utilizes measures obtained during standardized EDX testing and can be performed in any EMG laboratory. The NI is calculated as (CMAP amplitude/DML) $\times$ F – frequency %.[35] Compared with other clinical measures such as ALS Functional Rating Scale, forced vital capacity, CMAP amplitude and muscle strength, NI correlates well with ALS progression.[35,36] In addition, it has robust reproducibility and intrarater reliability and is sensitive for differentiating between rapidly and slowly progressive forms of ALS.[35]

Motor Unit Number Estimate

The MUNE is a quantitative measurement to evaluate available motor units. To calculate MUNE, the maximum CMAP amplitude is divided by the average amplitude of single MUPs. Over the years, different methods for single MUP estimation have been developed, making the test accurate and reproducible. MUNE is reliable for tracking motor neuron loss in ALS and, compared with CMAP, muscle strength, and forced vital capacity, is more sensitive to change with disease progression.[37]

Motor Unit Number Index

Similar to MUNE, but somewhat faster to record and calculate, the motor unit number index (MUNIX) provides reliable and reproducible quantitative information about relative change in number of motor units. Using a mathematical model, MUNIX is calculated using CMAP amplitude and surface EMG interference patterns. To obtain surface EMG interference pattern values, a surface EMG is recorded with the patient maintaining a brief isometric contraction at varying levels of force. The CMAP and these different surface EMG interference pattern epochs are analyzed by software to obtain the MUNIX. The motor unit size index can then be calculated, dividing CMAP by MUNIX. Both the motor unit size index and MUNIX reflect, but are not direct measurements of, the actual number of motor units or the size of individual motor units. Together, they are helpful for detecting early MUP loss in ALS, even when CMAP and muscle force remain relatively stable.[38,39]

Electrical Impedance Myography. EIM applies surface currents to measure the electrical impedance of underlying muscle tissue. EIM may help to diagnose and evaluate disease severity and progression in different neuromuscular disorders, including ALS. This technique allows flexibility in evaluating different body regions to track ALS progression and focuses the analysis on the most symptomatic body region.[40] Compared with other EDX methods with a limited ability to evaluate tongue function, EIM may allow a more detailed study of tongue dysfunction as ALS progresses.[41] EIM measures seem to correlate with other clinical measures, including revised the ALS Functional Rating Scale and handheld dynamometry, suggesting a possible future role as a marker of disease progression in ALS clinical trials.[40]

OTHER MOTOR NEURON DISEASES

Other chronic NMDs share many similarities with ALS in the abnormalities noted on EDX. The clinical presentation and EDX findings of some key disorders that may mimic ALS are reviewed, and differentiating EDX features are summarized in **Table 1**.

Primary Lateral Sclerosis and Progressive Muscular Atrophy

Both primary lateral sclerosis (PLS) and progressive muscular atrophy are degenerative MNDs that present later in life. They are less common than ALS. The initial symptoms can make them difficult to distinguish from ALS and there is debate as to whether they are distinct entities or exist along a spectrum with ALS.[42–45]

In PLS, there is progressive degeneration of cortical motor neurons without significant changes in the anterior horn cells.[44] The most common clinical manifestations include leg and bulbar spasticity and weakness.[44] In contrast with ALS, PLS is more often symmetric initially with a more indolent progression and a more benign clinical course. In general, NCS should be normal and EMG may show poor voluntary muscle activation, but should otherwise be normal. Occasional, patients with PLS may demonstrate mild signs of LMN dysfunction years after symptom onset, which may favor the reclassification of their disease as UMN-onset ALS.[44,45]

Progressive muscular atrophy is a disorder with progressive LMN degeneration without clinical UMN involvement. It generally starts focally in a distal limb with muscle atrophy, weakness, and fasciculations, and then spreads to contiguous regions. Patients with progressive muscular atrophy are typically younger than patients with ALS and have a longer survival from symptom onset, although those with axial involvement at symptom onset, or more profound denervation in the paraspinal muscles, are more likely to have early respiratory dysfunction and a worse prognosis.[46]

Spinal Muscular Atrophy

SMA is the most common cause of MND in the pediatric population. Most cases are secondary to homozygous mutation in the survival motor neuron 1 gene (SMN1), resulting in degeneration of LMNs, progressive muscle weakness, and atrophy. The severity of disease correlates with the number of copies of a related gene, SMN2; patients with infantile-onset SMA type 1 have the fewest SMN2 copies and young adult onset SMA type 4 have the most.[47] Milder forms of SMA occasionally may be mistaken for muscular dystrophy or other diseases, making EDX an important ancillary step in SMA diagnosis. EDX testing also provides another means for assessing improvement or stability with newer therapeutic interventions.

Table 1
Comparison of EDX features of other motor neuron disorders with ALS

	NCS	EMG	MUNE	RNS
Progressive muscular atrophy	a	a	a	a
Spinal muscular atrophy	CMAP decrease less profound and may plateau	Lower amplitude, fewer fibrillations Infrequent fasciculation potentials More CRDs and neuromyotonic discharges	Milder SMA type 2 and 3 may show increased MUNE, decreased SMUP from baseline	a
Spinobulbar muscular atrophy	CMAP decrease is less profound SNAPs decreased	Simpler fasciculation morphology	a	a
Hirayama disease	CMAP reduction mainly in hand	More stable MUP	a	Not reported
Post-polio syndrome	CMAP decrease is less profound	Larger, more stable MUPs	Less progressive decline	

Abbreviations: CMAP, compound muscle action potentials; CRD, complex repetitive discharges; EMG, electromyography; MUNE, motor unit number estimate; MUP, motor unit potentials; NCS, nerve conduction studies; RNS, repetitive nerve stimulation; SMUP, single motor unit potential.
a = findings similar to ALS (individual variations exist and findings depend on disease severity).

Spinal Bulbar Muscular Atrophy

Spinal bulbar muscular atrophy, or Kennedy disease, is an X-linked recessive disorder secondary to a trinucleotide CAG repeat expansion in the androgen gene. It is a slowly progressive MND that mainly affects the bulbar and spinal motor neurons and is associated with testicular atrophy, gynecomastia, and sensory neuropathy. It can mimic ALS with slow progression.[48] Sensory nerve action potentials are frequently low amplitude in spinal bulbar muscular atrophy.

Hirayama Disease

Hirayama disease or unilateral upper extremity juvenile muscular atrophy occurs primarily in males and is characterized by unilateral slowly progressive muscle weakness and wasting of the hand and forearm that spontaneously arrest after several years.[49] Neuropathology and neuroimaging studies have shown evidence of anteroposterior flattening and ischemic necrotic changes in the anterior horn cells of the cervical spinal cord, especially in the C7 to C8 region, as well as shifting of the posterior dural sac and engorgement of the posterior epidural venous plexus. The cause of Hirayama disease is unclear, but in many cases is thought to be related to chronic cervical spinal cord injury secondary to ischemia or compression from cervical spine flexion. Other proposed mechanisms include autoimmune and genetic factors.[49,50] Needle EMG demonstrates neurogenic changes in the C7 to C8 muscles, sparing the C5 to C6 muscles.

Postpolio Syndrome

Poliomyelitis is a monophasic viral infection resulting in localized or generalized LMN loss. However, for some patients the neurologic deterioration may progress years after the initial insult. Patients with postpolio syndrome may experience decreased muscle strength up to 2.5% yearly.[51] In addition to the loss of whole motor units, partial loss of distal axons in enlarged motor units late in disease compounds underlying ineffective reinnervation to cause decreased strength.[51]

SUMMARY

When MNDs are suspected, NCS, conventional needle EMG, SF EMG, and RNS can all demonstrate abnormalities that help with diagnosis and exclude other causes. Among these measures, increased jitter, decrement on a 2-Hz RNS, and unstable units on needle EMG are concerning for a worse prognosis in ALS. Newer techniques, including MUNE, MUNIX, and NI, are more sensitive for early ALS detection. However, especially with MUNE and MUNIX, their usefulness is limited owing to technical challenges. Although many EDX similarities are observed across all motor neuron disorders, pathophysiological differences do give rise to distinguishing EDX features with each disorder.

CLINICS CARE POINTS

- EDX study is crucial for the accurate diagnosis in patients with MND and helps to exclude other conditions in the differential diagnosis.

- NCS testing of patients with ALS may demonstrate decreased CMAP amplitudes, mild DML prolongation, less persistent F-wave responses, and decremental response on slow RNS. Sensory NCS testing occasionally may be mildly abnormal.

- FPs and fibrillation potentials are widespread and prominent in ALS. Unstable MUP morphology and increased jitter are concerning for poor prognosis.

- NI, MUNE, and MUNIX can detect early changes in ALS. However, the usefulness of MUNE and MUNIX are limited owing to technical and other factors.

> • Progressive muscular atrophy, SMA, spinal bulbar muscular atrophy, Hirayama disease and PPS are other diseases involving localized or generalized LMN degeneration. There are EDX features associated with each that help to distinguish these conditions from ALS.

DISCLOSURE

Dr X. Kang has no disclosures; Dr D. Quan has received funding from the following entities to perform clinical research: Alnylam, Pfizer, Cytokinetics, Argenx, Momenta, Alexion, Ionis Viela Bio, Apellis; Dr D. Quan has received consulting fees from Alnylam.

REFERENCES

1. Daube JR. Electrophysiologic studies in the diagnosis and prognosis of motor neuron diseases. Neurol Clin 1985;3:8.
2. Daube JR. Electrodiagnostic studies in amyotrophic lateral sclerosis and other motor neuron disorders. Muscle Nerve 2000;23(10):1488–502.
3. Tiryaki E, Horak H. ALS and Other motor neuron diseases. Continuum (Minneap Minn) 2014;20:1185–207.
4. Foster LA, Salajegheh MK. Motor neuron disease: pathophysiology, diagnosis and management. Am J Med 2019;132:32–7.
5. Kincaid O, Lipton HL. Viral myelitis: an update. Curr Neurol Neurosci Rep 2006; 6(6):469.
6. Bitnun A, Yeh EA. Acute flaccid paralysis and enteroviral infections. Curr Infect Dis Rep 2018;20(9):34.
7. AANEM Nomenclature Committee. AANEM Glossary of Terms in Neuromuscular and Electrodiagnostic Medicine, Muscle and Nerve Supplement 2015. S1.
8. Chiò A, Logroscino G, Traynor BJ, et al. Global epidemiology of amyotrophic lateral sclerosis: a systematic review of the published literature. Neuroepidemiology 2013;41(2):118–30.
9. Kent-Braun JA, Walker CH, Weiner MW, et al. Functional significance of upper and lower motor neuron impairment in amyotrophic lateral sclerosis. Muscle Nerve 1998;21(6):762–8.
10. de Carvalho M, Chio A, Dengler R, et al. Neurophysiological measures in amyotrophic lateral sclerosis: markers of progression in clinical trials. Amyotroph Lateral Scler Other Motor Neuron Disord 2005;6(1):17–28.
11. de Carvalho M, Swash M. Nerve conduction studies in amyotrophic lateral sclerosis. Muscle Nerve 2000;23(3):344–52.
12. Brooks BR, Miller RG, Swash M, et al. World Federation of Neurology Research Group on Motor Neuron Diseases. El Escorial revisited: revised criteria for the diagnosis of amyotrophic lateral sclerosis. Amyotroph Lateral Scler Other Motor Neuron Disord 2000;1(5):293–9.
13. de Carvalho M, Dengler R, Eisen A, et al. Electrodiagnostic criteria for diagnosis of ALS. Clin Neurophysiol 2008;119(3):497–503.
14. Wang FC, Delwaide PJ. Number and relative size of thenar motor units in ALS patients: application of the adapted multiple point stimulation method. Electroencephalogr Clin Neurophysiol 1998;109(1):36–43.
15. Ertaş M, Uludağ B, Ertekin C. Slow motor conduction mainly limited to motor root in amyotrophic lateral sclerosis. Muscle Nerve 1996;19(8):1003–8.
16. Eisen A, Swash M. Clinical neurophysiology of ALS. Clin Neurophysiol 2001; 112(12):2190–201.

17. Lange DJ, Trojaborg W, McDonald TD, et al. Persistent and transient "conduction block" in motor neuron diseases. Muscle Nerve 1993;16(9):896–903.

18. Mills KR, Nithi KA. Peripheral and central motor conduction in amyotrophic lateral sclerosis. J Neurol Sci 1998;159(1):82–7.

19. Chaudhry V, Clawson LL. Entrapment of motor nerves in motor neuron disease: does double crush occur? J Neurol Neurosurg Psychiatry 1997;62(1):71–6.

20. Simon NG, Lomen-Hoerth C, Kiernan MC. Patterns of clinical and electrodiagnostic abnormalities in early amyotrophic lateral sclerosis. Muscle Nerve 2014;50(6):894–9.

21. Schelhaas HJ, van de Warrenburg BP, Kremer HP, et al. The "split hand" phenomenon: evidence of a spinal origin. Neurology 2003;61(11):1619–20.

22. Isak B, Tankisi H, Johnsen B, et al. Involvement of distal sensory nerves in amyotrophic lateral sclerosis. Muscle Nerve 2016;54(6):1086–92.

23. Hammad M, Silva A, Glass J, et al. Clinical, electrophysiologic, and pathologic evidence for sensory abnormalities in ALS. Neurology 2007;69(24):2236–42.

24. de Carvalho M, Swash M. Fasciculation potentials and earliest changes in motor unit physiology in ALS. J Neurol Neurosurg Psychiatry 2013;84(9):963–8.

25. de Carvalho M, Turkman A, Swash M. Sensitivity of MUP parameters in detecting change in early ALS. Clin Neurophysiol 2014;125(1):166–9.

26. de Carvalho M, Swash M. Fasciculation discharge frequency in amyotrophic lateral sclerosis and related disorders. Clin Neurophysiol 2016;127(5):2257–62.

27. Wang FC, De Pasqua V, Gérard P, et al. Prognostic value of decremental responses to repetitive nerve stimulation in ALS patients. Neurology 2001;57(5):897–9.

28. Iwanami T, Sonoo M, Hatanaka Y, et al. Decremental responses to repetitive nerve stimulation (RNS) in motor neuron disease. Clin Neurophysiol 2011;122(12):2530–6.

29. Zhang D, Zhao Y, Yan C, et al. CMAP decrement by low-frequency repetitive nerve stimulation in different hand muscles of ALS patients. Neurol Sci 2019;40(12):2609–15.

30. de Carvalho M, Swash M. The split hand in amyotrophic lateral sclerosis: a possible role for the neuromuscular junction. Amyotroph Lateral Scler Frontotemporal Degener 2019;20(5–6):368–75.

31. Inoue K, Hemmi S, Miyaishi M, et al. Muscular fatigue and decremental response to repetitive nerve stimulation in X-linked spinobulbar muscular atrophy. Eur J Neurol 2009;16(1):76–80.

32. Wadman RI, Vrancken AF, van den Berg LH, et al. Dysfunction of the neuromuscular junction in spinal muscular atrophy types 2 and 3. Neurology 2012;79(20):2050–5.

33. Zheng C, Jin X, Zhu Y, et al. Repetitive nerve stimulation as a diagnostic aid for distinguishing cervical spondylotic amyotrophy from amyotrophic lateral sclerosis. Eur Spine J 2017;26(7):1929–36.

34. Liu M, Cui L, Guan Y, et al. Single-fiber electromyography in amyotrophic lateral sclerosis and cervical spondylosis. Muscle Nerve 2013;48(1):137–9.

35. Swash M, de Carvalho M. The Neurophysiological Index in ALS. Amyotroph Lateral Scler Other Motor Neuron Disord 2004;5(Suppl 1):108–10.

36. de Carvalho M, Swash M. Sensitivity of electrophysiological tests for upper and lower motor neuron dysfunction in ALS: a six-month longitudinal study. Muscle Nerve 2010;41(2):208–11.

37. Gooch CL, Doherty TJ, Chan KM, et al. Motor unit number estimation: a technology and literature review. Muscle Nerve 2014;50(6):884–93.

38. Escorcio-Bezerra ML, Abrahao A, Nunes KF, et al. Motor unit number index and neurophysiological index as candidate biomarkers of presymptomatic motor neuron loss in amyotrophic lateral sclerosis. Muscle Nerve 2018;58(2):204–12.
39. Nandedkar SD, Barkhaus PE, Stålberg EV. Motor unit number index (MUNIX): principle, method, and findings in healthy subjects and in patients with motor neuron disease. Muscle Nerve 2010;42(5):798–807.
40. Rutkove SB, Caress JB, Cartwright MS, et al. Electrical impedance myography correlates with standard measures of ALS severity. Muscle Nerve 2014;49(3): 441–3.
41. Shellikeri S, Yunusova Y, Green JR, et al. Electrical impedance myography in the evaluation of the tongue musculature in amyotrophic lateral sclerosis. Muscle Nerve 2015;52(4):584–91.
42. Sorenson EJ. The electrophysiology of the motor neuron diseases. Neurol Clin 2012;30(2):605–20.
43. Ince PG, Evans J, Knopp M, et al. Corticospinal tract degeneration in the progressive muscular atrophy variant of ALS. Neurology 2003;60(8):1252–8.
44. Statland JM, Barohn RJ, Dimachkie MM, et al. Primary lateral sclerosis. Neurol Clin 2015;33(4):749–60.
45. Singer MA, Kojan S, Barohn RJ, et al. Primary lateral sclerosis: clinical and laboratory features in 25 patients. J Clin Neuromuscul Dis 2005;7(1):1–9.
46. de Carvalho M, Scotto M, Swash M. Clinical patterns in progressive muscular atrophy (PMA): a prospective study. Amyotroph Lateral Scler 2007;8(5):296–9.
47. Wadman RI, Stam M, Gijzen M, et al. Association of motor milestones, SMN2 copy and outcome in spinal muscular atrophy types 0-4. J Neurol Neurosurg Psychiatry 2017;88(4):365–7.
48. Parboosingh JS, Figlewicz DA, Krizus A, et al. Spinobulbar muscular atrophy can mimic ALS: the importance of genetic testing in male patients with atypical ALS. Neurology 1997;49(2):568–72.
49. Hirayama K. [Juvenile muscular atrophy of unilateral upper extremity (Hirayama disease)–half-century progress and establishment since its discovery]. Brain Nerve 2008;60(1):17–29.
50. Kira J, Ochi H. Juvenile muscular atrophy of the distal upper limb (Hirayama disease) associated with atopy. J Neurol Neurosurg Psychiatry 2001;70(6):798–801.
51. Bickerstaffe A, van Dijk JP, Beelen A, et al. Loss of motor unit size and quadriceps strength over 10 years in post-polio syndrome. Clin Neurophysiol 2014;125(6): 1255–60.

Electrodiagnostic Assessment of Hyperexcitable Nerve Disorders

Spencer K. Hutto, MD, Taylor B. Harrison, MD*

KEYWORDS

- Peripheral nerve hyperexcitability • Myokymia • Neuromyotonia • Isaacs syndrome
- Morvan syndrome • Cramp-fasciculation syndrome • VGKC-complex antibodies

KEY POINTS

- Peripheral nerve hyperexcitability (PNH) constitutes a variety of disorders along an electroclinical spectrum of cramps, fasciculations, myokymia, neuromyotonia, dysautonomia, and encephalopathy.
- Disorders of PNH include cramp-fasciculation syndrome, Isaacs syndrome, and Morvan syndrome. Myokymia, neuromyotonia, and dysautonomia are features of both Isaacs and Morvan syndromes, and central nervous system dysfunction is a defining characteristic of Morvan syndrome.
- Sensitivity of detecting myokymia and neuromyotonia on needle electromyography in Isaacs and Morvan syndromes increases with sampling of distal muscles.
- Patients with myokymia or neuromyotonia associated with leucine-rich glioma-inactivated 1 (LGI1) or contactin-associated protein-2 (CASPR2) antibodies may have an underlying neoplasm.

INTRODUCTION

The syndromes of peripheral nerve hyperexcitability (PNH) are relatively rare disorders characterized by involuntary muscle twitching, cramping, and muscle stiffness. Other symptoms include exercise intolerance, hyperhidrosis, mood irritability, insomnia, and encephalopathy. Characteristic electrodiagnostic (EDX) findings include fasciculation potentials, cramp potentials, myokymia, and neuromyotonia. Over the years, numerous investigators proposed several descriptive and eponymous names for PNH syndrome.[1,2] This article focuses on 3 PNH disorders: cramp-fasciculation syndrome (CFS), Issacs syndrome, and Morvan syndrome, recognizing that core clinical and EDX features differentiate these clinical entities (**Fig. 1**).

Department of Neurology, Emory University School of Medicine, 12 Executive Park Drive Northeast, Room 150H, Atlanta, GA 30329, USA
* Corresponding author.
E-mail address: tharri4@emory.edu

Neurol Clin 39 (2021) 1083–1096
https://doi.org/10.1016/j.ncl.2021.06.009
0733-8619/21/© 2021 Elsevier Inc. All rights reserved.

	CFS	Isaacs	Morvan
Male Preponderance	X	X	XXX
Cramps/Fasciculations	X	X	X
Myokymia/NMT on EDX		X	X
Dysautonomia		X	XX
CNS Dysfunction			X
Cancer		X	XX
Neural Autoantibodies	X	XX	XXX

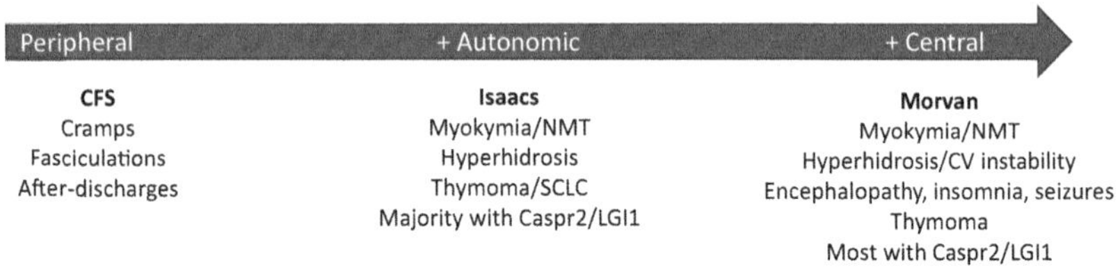

Peripheral	+ Autonomic	+ Central
CFS	**Isaacs**	**Morvan**
Cramps	Myokymia/NMT	Myokymia/NMT
Fasciculations	Hyperhidrosis	Hyperhidrosis/CV instability
After-discharges	Thymoma/SCLC	Encephalopathy, insomnia, seizures
	Majority with Caspr2/LGI1	Thymoma
		Most with Caspr2/LGI1

Fig. 1. Comparison of clinical and EDX features of cardinal disorders of PNH.

HISTORY

Disorders of PNH first were described approximately 130 years ago when, in 1890, Augustin Morvan first reported on his eponym of mixed peripheral nervous system (PNS) and central nervous system (CNS) dysfunction when he described 5 patients with "fibrillary chorea," referring to the apparent dancing of muscle fibers underneath the skin in patients.[3] These patients also demonstrated signs of autonomic dysfunction, fluctuating encephalopathy, and insomnia. In the ensuing decades, sparse reports of similar cases ensued (reviewed by Serratrice and Azulay[4]). The original description of the second syndrome of PNH was published 1961, wherein Hyam Issacs[5] coined a term for a syndrome of "continuous muscle fiber activity" (subsequently referred to as Isaacs syndrome) in 2 patients who presented with gradually progressive generalized muscle stiffness with muscle twitching and hyperhidrosis. Isaacs syndrome is phenotypically different from Morvan syndrome due to the absence of CNS symptomatology (including insomnia, hallucinations, personality change, and encephalopathy). The final major manifestation of PNH was described in 1991 by Tahmoush and colleagues,[6] who described a milder syndrome of myalgia, cramps, stiffness, and exercise intolerance in what they called CFS.

ELECTRODIAGNOSTIC FINDINGS IN PERIPHERAL NERVE HYPEREXCITABILITY

The classic EDX abnormalities seen in PNH constitute abnormal insertional and spontaneous motor unit activity noted on needle electromyography (EMG). Volitional motor unit morphology and recruitment generally are normal unless there is an underlying neuromuscular condition contributing to secondary PNH. A diverse array of discharges has been described, including (1) fasciculations, (2) cramp potentials, (3) myokymic discharges, and (4) neuromyotonic discharges.[7] Nerve conduction studies (NCSs) may show abnormal afterdischarges (ADs) after routine motor NCSs, with assessment of late responses, such as F-responses and H-reflexes, and after repetitive nerve stimulation (RNS).

Fasciculation Potentials

Fasciculations present clinically as irregular muscle twitching, which may be observed when superficial muscle fibers are activated by the spontaneous depolarization of a motor axon. This twitching does not cause movement across a joint, and fasciculations involving deeper regions of muscle or under thick subcutaneous tissue may be identified only by needle examination. Denny-Brown and Pennybacker[8] first described the fasciculation potential in 1938 as the spontaneous discharge of an individual motor unit, which constitutes an anterior horn cell, its associated axon, and all the muscle fibers it innervates. The source generator of this discharge is the motor nerve or the axon terminal, in spite of the classic association of these discharges with diseases of the anterior horn cell.[9,10] On needle examination, fasciculation potentials fire erratically. The irregular and typically slow firing pattern requires patience, because fasciculations may be missed if an examiner is rushed during the examination. When multiple fasciculations are noted, the morphology of each fasciculation potential typically is variable because different potentials reflect spontaneous activation of different motor units (**Fig. 2**). Most fasciculation potentials have normal motor unit morphology for the muscle from which they are recorded, unless there is an underlying neuromuscular disorder associated with chronic reinnervation changes.

Cramp Potentials

Cramps manifest clinically as painful and palpable muscle tightening (of a single muscle) that is relieved by stretching. Cramps are common among the general population and generally associated with electrolyte derangements, dehydration, and multiple medications.[11] The generator of a cramp potential historically is the motor unit, although there is some evidence that the distal motor unit, in particular the intramuscular nerve terminals, constitutes the predominant source generator.[10] Cramps typically are associated with muscle activation (eg, exercise) but may be spontaneous. In isolation they are nonspecific for cause but in the setting of muscle twitching and muscle stiffness cramps may herald PNH.

On EMG, muscle cramps are composed of continuous motor unit potentials (MUPs) firing at frequencies up to 150 Hz. During the evolution of a cramp discharge, the frequency of firing and amplitude of the discharge increase and then slowly subside.[10,12] They typically are preceded by recurrent fasciculations, which also may be observed after cessation of the cramp discharge. Stimulus-induced cramp discharges also may be recorded with surface electrodes and identified when the frequency of ADs increases such that individual ADs cannot be identified (**Fig. 3**).

Myokymia

The EDX features of myokymic discharges first were described in 1948 by Denny-Brown and Foley.[13] Myokymia is a descriptive term stemming from the clinical observation of undulating movement of the overlying skin or mucous membranes (eg, the tongue) as a result of spontaneous repetitive discharges from 2 or more motor

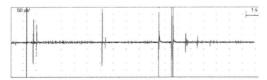

Fig. 2. Multiple fasciculation potentials are depicted on this tracing. Note the slow sweep speed of 1 s/division. (*Adapted from* Rubin DI. Normal and abnormal spontaneous activity. Handb Clin Neurol. 2019;160:257-279; with permission.)

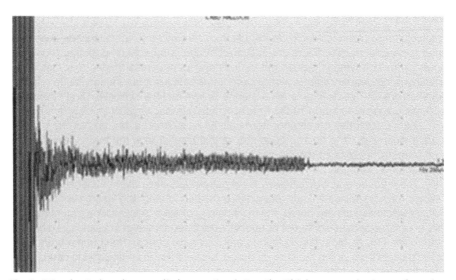

Fig. 3. Stimulus-induced cramp discharge stimulating the tibial nerve and using surface electrodes over abductor hallucis brevis. Note onset of cramp potential is immediately after stimulation and innumerable Ads contribute to the waveform. Sweep speed is 1 s/division and gain is 100 μV/division. (*From* Benatar M, Chapman KM, Rutkove SB. Repetitive nerve stimulation for the evaluation of peripheral nerve hyperexcitability. J Neurol Sci. 2004;221(1-2):47-52; with permission.)

units.[9,12] Although myokymia can be observed clinically, this not always is the case, particularly when the affected muscle is deep either within the bulk of muscle or under deep subcutaneous tissue.

Double, triple, and multiple discharges reflect the spontaneous firing of 2 or more MUPs of similar morphology and amplitude that occur in a similar sequence during each burst.[12] The interval between each discharge usually is in the range of 2 milliseconds (ms) to 20 ms, with the duration between the second and third action potentials often exceeding that between the first 2 (**Fig. 4**). The generator is the motor unit or motor axon and essentially synonymous with fasciculation potentials. They can be thought of as grouped fasciculations, classically associated with tetany from hypocalcemia or hypomagnesemia, which is important to consider in the differential diagnosis.[14]

Myokymic discharges occur most typically as double or multiple discharges (up to 10) with rhythmic or semirhythmic bursts, typically described as the sound of marching soldiers.[12,14] These spontaneous bursts cycle as a group between bursts and silence. The intraburst (within the burst) frequency (5–60 Hz) is faster than the interburst (between-burst) frequency, which typically is 2 Hz or less. There is much variability on burst morphology and both intraburst and interburst frequency, because myokymic discharges can contain bursts of more than 100 motor units and burst frequency as slow as every 20 s[15] (**Fig. 5**).

Myokymic discharges can be localized (focal) or generalized, the latter typically associated with disorders of PNH. Focal myokymia may be restricted to facial musculature, 1 limb, or the distribution of a spinal root or motor nerve. There are multiple causes of focal myokymia (**Box 1**).[16] Myokymia can be confused with other spontaneous discharges, such as complex repetitive discharges or tremor (**Table 1**).

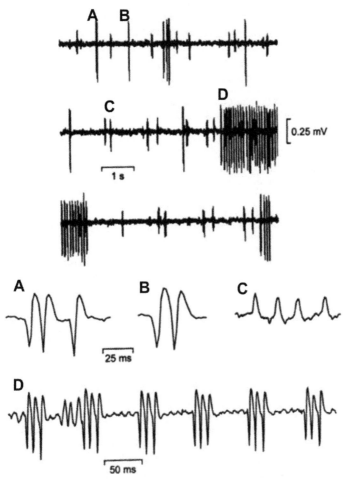

Fig. 4. Upper trace is a 25-s continuous needle EMG recording from medial gastrocnemius. Different motor units are seen to fire spontaneously and irregularly as double discharges (B), triple discharges (A), and multiple discharges (C), with intraburst frequencies of up to 120 Hz. The prolonged discharge in the middle of the recording consists of rapidly firing triple discharges of more than 1 motor unit (D). (*From* Maddison P, Mills KR, Newsom-Davis J. Clinical electrophysiological characterization of the acquired neuromyotonia phenotype of autoimmune peripheral nerve hyperexcitability. Muscle Nerve. 2006;33(6):801-808; with permission.)

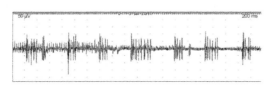

Fig. 5. Schematic of myokymic discharge. Sweep speed is 200 ms/division and gain is 50 μV/division. (*From* Rubin DI. Normal and abnormal spontaneous activity. Handb Clin Neurol. 2019;160:257-279; with permission.)

Box 1
Disorders associated with focal and generalized myokymia

Facial
  Pontine lesions (multiple sclerosis, glioma, and others)
  Cerebellopontine angle masses (schwannomas)
  Vascular compression (basilar invagination)
  Facial neuropathies (Bell's palsy, Guillain-Barré syndrome, sarcoidosis, and basilar meningitis)
  Motor neuron disease (eg, Kennedy disease)

Regional
  Myelopathy
  Radiculopathy (structural or demyelinating)
  Plexopathy (eg, postradiation injury)
  Mononeuropathy (compressive or traumatic)

Generalized
  PNH syndromes (Isaacs and Morvan syndromes)
  Hereditary diseases (episodic ataxia type 1, axonal neuropathy with neuromyotonia, and Charcot-Marie-Tooth disease)
  Acquired demyelinating neuropathies (acute and chronic acquired demyelinating polyneuropathies)Motor neuron diseases (amyotrophic lateral sclerosis)
  Toxic exposures (heavy metals, penicillamine, and timber rattlesnake envenomation)
  Thyrotoxicosis

Adapted from Katirji B. Peripheral nerve hyperexcitability. Handb Clin Neurol. 2019;161:281-290; with permission.

Neuromyotonia

The EDX features of neuromyotonia originally were described in 1965 by Mertens and Zschocke.[17] Neuromyotonic discharges are very high frequency (150–300 Hz) bursts of MUPs that wane in amplitude throughout the burst and start/stop abruptly, either spontaneously or as a result of needle movement or voluntary contraction[12] (**Fig. 6**).

Clinically, neuromyotonia is manifest as persistent muscle contraction.[18] Some investigators posit that myokymic and neuromyotonic discharges exist along a frequency spectrum but have the same significance.[18] Neuromyotonia constitutes a more specific finding for PNH, because myokymia is associated with more diverse pathologic entities, as discussed previously.

Afterdischarges

ADs are repetitive or sustained firing of action potentials that occur after stimulation and persist beyond stimulus cessation. ADs have been noted after routine motor NCSs and during late responses in patients with PNH.[19–23] In the setting of F-waves, ADs may obscure the late response (**Fig. 7**). A gain of 200 μV and a time base of 20 ms/division may facilitate the identification of ADs during routine motor NCSs (**Fig. 8**).[20,24]

RNS has been proposed as potentially useful for identifying stimulus-induced ADs with surface electrodes. Various studies have reported the identification of abnormal ADs, many of which reported qualitive data about the presence or absence of ADs.[6,25,26] Various recording setups have been utilized, with a sweep speed of 100 ms–1 s/division and a gain of 100 μV/division to 200 μV/division most commonly reported. Because the distal axon and motor end plate are suspected to contribute to the generation of the spontaneous discharges in PNH, distal stimulation is performed in a standard fashion for routine motor NCSs. The tibial nerve may provide optimal sensitivity and specificity, concordant with reports noting neuromyotonia and

Table 1			
Myokymia mimics			
EMG Discharge	**Source Generator**	**Morphology**	**Firing Characteristics**
Myokymia	Motor unit	Looks like grouped fasciculations, on speaker sounds like marching solders. Number of intraburst potentials may vary.	Intraburst (within-burst) frequency of 5–60 Hz Interburst (between-burst) frequency of 2 Hz or less
Complex repetitive discharge	Muscle fiber, with ephaptic spread to adjacent fibers	Regular, high frequency (20–150 Hz) polyspike discharge. Morphology may change due to drop out or additional involvement of nearby muscle fibers. Machine-like sound on amplifier.	Begins and stops abruptly
Tremor	Central cause stimulates a variable population of anterior horn cells	Motor units within each burst vary	Interburst frequency of 4–19 Hz depending on cause of tremor (Parkinson disease, essential tremor, orthostatic tremor)

myokymia are more prominent distally than proximally and more prominent in the legs than arms.[22,26] Various stimulation frequencies have been employed, ranging from 1 Hz to 30 Hz, with sensitivity optimized at high RNS rates and specificity improved with low stimulation frequencies.[25,26] It is important to be careful to not misinterpret voluntary muscle activation or impaired relaxation on surface EMG as being indicative of PNH.

The clinical relevance of ADs, particularly with regard to ADs provoked by RNS, is questionable. Evaluation of ADs in normal controls and patients with polyneuropathy

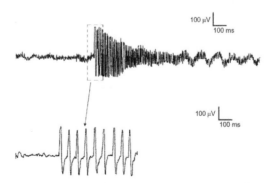

100 µV
100 ms

100 µV
100 ms

Fig. 6. Neuromyotonic discharge. Note the decrementing response. The top is recorded with a long sweep speed of 100 ms/division while the insert is at a regular sweep speed of 10 ms/division. Note the very-high-frequency (150–250 Hz) repetitive discharge of a single motor unit. (*From* Preston DC, Shapiro BE. (2013). Electromyography and neuromuscular disorders, third edition. London: Elsevier/Saunders; with permission.)

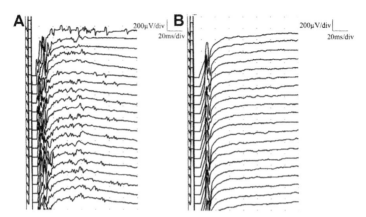

Fig. 7. Prolonged ADs noted after median f-responses, note the ADs obscure the median f responses. (*From* Niu J, Guan H, Cui L, Guan Y, Liu M. Afterdischarges following M waves in patients with voltage-gated potassium channels antibodies. Clin Neurophysiol Pract. 2017;2:72-75; with permission.)

has failed to identify differences in AD duration between groups.[27] Furthermore, the average duration of stimulus-induced ADs following stimulation at various frequencies (between 2 Hz and 20 Hz) in patients with CFS with and without voltage-gated potassium channels (VGKCs) antibodies did not discriminate between seropositive and seronegative patients.[28] Thus, RNS-induced ADs in patients undergoing evaluation for CFS should be interpreted cautiously, given the common presence of ADs in the normal population and apparent lack of specificity.[27,29] More information is needed regarding the typical duration of ADs in the normal population and the prevalence of

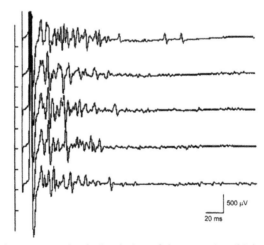

Fig. 8. ADs following supramaximal stimulation of the posterior tibial nerve; 5 consecutive compound muscle action potentials are followed directly by trains of asynchronous ADs. (*From* Maddison P, Mills KR, Newsom-Davis J. Clinical electrophysiological characterization of the acquired neuromyotonia phenotype of autoimmune peripheral nerve hyperexcitability. Muscle Nerve. 2006;33(6):801-808; with permission.)

ADs in common neuromuscular diseases to determine if ADs can discriminate between those with and without CFS.[27]

THE CLINICAL SPECTRUM OF PERIPHERAL NERVE HYPEREXCITABILITY

The causes of PNH are myriad and largely can be divided into primary (presumed autoimmune, paraneoplastic, or hereditary) and secondary etiologies (related to varied pathology affecting motor nerves or neurons). Conceptually, disorders of PNH can be considered to lie along an electroclinical spectrum with more benign disease typically limited to the PNS, as in CFS, and more severe disease associated with additional dysfunction of the CNS and autonomic nervous system (ANS), as in Isaacs and Morvan syndromes. The presence of an associated neural autoantibody becomes increasingly more likely as abnormal spontaneous activity is seen on EMG or when CNS or ANS dysfunction are apparent. A proportion of patients are found to have a paraneoplastic disorder, with thymoma, non–small cell lung carcinoma, and thyroid cancer the most commonly associated neoplasms.[30–32] Hereditary causes of PNH include episodic ataxia type 1 and axonal neuropathy with neuromyotonia.[33,34]

PNS hyperexcitability commonly is ascribed to dysfunction of VGKCs, which function to repolarize the nerve and, in disease, reduce the threshold to nerve depolarization.[35] The association of PNH with VGKC-complex antibodies first was suspected by Newsom-Davis and Mills in 1993.[36] The specific antigens were later clarified to be associated with the VGKC-complex rather than the actual channel (**Fig. 9**).[36,37] Contactin-associated protein 2 (Caspr2) is involved in the clustering of potassium channels at the juxtaparanodal region on myelinated axons and also is found centrally in the cerebellum and hippocampus.[38] Leucine-rich glioma-inactivated 1 (LGI1) modulates synaptic transmission and is expressed mainly in the hippocampus and temporal cortex, hence its association with limbic encephalitis and faciobrachial dystonic seizures (FBDS).[37] Although Caspr2 is associated more commonly with Isaacs and Morvan syndromes and LGI1 with limbic encephalitis and FBDS, the clinical

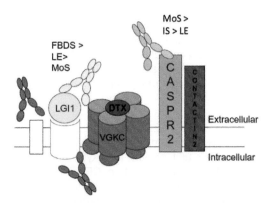

Fig. 9. Depiction of the VGKC-complex labeled with dendrotoxin (DTX), the snake neurotoxin that binds strongly to VGKC, to show antibodies known to bind the extracellular domains of LGI1 (in patients with limbic encephalitis [LE], FBDS, and Morvan syndrome [MoS]), and Caspr2 in patients with MoS more frequently than in Issacs syndrome (IS) or LE. Contactin-2 antibodies are rare. Some antibodies may bind the intracellular domains of some molecules within the VGKC-complex (blue antibody). (*Modified from* Irani SR, Vincent A. Voltage-gated potassium channel-complex autoimmunity and associated clinical syndromes. Handb Clin Neurol. 2016;133:185-197; with permission.)

phenotypes associated with these autoantibodies overlap considerably, and both are capable of causing PNS as well as CNS pathology.[35,39] Antibodies against components of the cell-surface VGKC-complex may interfere with this function in a variety of ways: modulating channel activity, channel cross-linking and internalization, and complement-mediated destruction.[39–41]

As a group, men are affected more commonly with PNH than are women, and the male preponderance increases greatly if neural autoantibodies or CNS features are present (93% male in Morvan syndrome). Morvan patients tend to be older (median age of 57) whereas those with CFS and Isaacs are most commonly in their 40s.[2,28,42]

When a patient presents with symptoms and signs compatible with PNH, routine sensory and motor nerve conductions should be performed in at least 1 symptomatic limb, with at least 2 limbs preferred. Motor responses as well as late responses should be reviewed carefully for ADs. EMG should focus on at least 1 symptomatic limb, sampling both proximal and distal musculature, as well as another limb to determine whether there is a regional or generalized pattern of PNH. EDX abnormalities may fluctuate over time, which emphasizes importance of repeat EDX testing in patients with worsened clinical symptoms and/or signs in spite of having a previously unremarkable examination.[2]

Cramp-Fasciculation Syndrome

With manifestations restricted to peripheral motor nerves, CFS is considered the least severe phenotype of PNH. Muscle cramps, twitching, muscle stiffness, and exercise intolerance are symptoms commonly reported.[6,25] Although weakness may be a reported symptom, weakness rarely is found on examination. Cramps may be induced or exacerbated by exercise or muscle activation, which is common among all disorders of PNH. Sensory symptoms also may be present, typically in the setting of an underlying polyneuropathy. Besides fasciculations, the examination otherwise is normal unless CFS is secondary to an underlying neuromuscular condition, such as polyneuropathy or radiculopathy. CFS phenotypically is different from Isaacs and Morvan syndromes because neuromyotonia and myokymia are not noted on EMG and CNS and ANS symptoms or signs are absent.

Routine motor and sensory NCSs should be conducted to exclude baseline disease of the nerve. Stimulus-induced ADs or cramps on RNS and fasciculation potentials on EMG can be seen, noting that the role of RNS-induced ADs and cramps are unclear at this time.[6] Neural antibodies (mostly against the VGKC-complex) are relatively uncommon, ranging from 16% to 32%, and rarely in association with tumor which is most commonly thymoma (in 6%).[28,30]

Isaacs Syndrome

The additional findings of dysautonomia, clinical myokymia, and EDX evidence of abnormal spontaneous motor unit activity (myokymic and/or neuromyotonic discharges) help differentiate Isaacs syndrome from CFS.[22] Hyperhidrosis is the primary dysautonomia, although other less common forms have been described, including dysphagia, sialorrhea, piloerection, and tachycardia.[16] Some investigators have posited that hyperhidrosis reflects the metabolic impact of continuous motor unit activity as opposed to true dysautonomia. The neurologic examination may reveal fasciculations and myokymia, pseudomyotonia (impaired relaxation after muscle activation), and hypertrophied muscles (most commonly affecting the calves, likely from continuous motor unit activity). Trousseau sign (carpopedal spasm caused by inflating the blood-pressure cuff to a level above systolic pressure for 3 minutes) and Chvostek sign (twitching of the facial muscles in response to tapping over the facial nerve) have been reported but appear to be uncommon. It is not uncommon for patients to complain of pain, which can be diffuse and tends to be length-dependent (eg, worse in the legs than the arms).[43]

Neuromyotonic discharges are more common in distal than proximal muscles and more commonly are in the legs than the arms.[2,22] In a study of autoimmune neuromyotonia associated with VGKC-complex antibodies, the most frequently seen findings on EMG were double, triple, or multiple discharges of high intraburst frequency (between 40 Hz and 350 Hz) in at least 1 symptomatic muscle.[22] VGKC-complex antibodies are present in up to half of cases (54%), ganglionic acetylcholine receptor antibodies in a minority (14%), and 1 or both in 63%. Thymoma and small cell lung cancer are the most commonly associated tumors; 16% of cases are paraneoplastic.[30] Issacs syndrome can be associated as a comorbid autoimmune phenomenon with myasthenia gravis and if the appropriate clinical history and examination are elicited, further evaluation for myasthenia is warranted.

Morvan Syndrome

In addition to the PNH stigmata seen in Isaacs syndrome, Morvan patients with Morvan syndrome typically have prominent sleep disturbances (insomnia, dream-enactment, and daytime hypersomnolence), a fluctuating encephalopathy, and vivid hallucinations.[19] Personality change with anxiety and agitation may be reported. Limb paresthesias and pain as well as skin lesions and pruritis are common.[19,42,43] Hyperhidrosis (86.2%) and cardiovascular instability (48.3%) are the most common dysautonomias.[19] Seizures and cerebellar dysfunction are present in one-third and weight loss in one-half.[42]

The primary approach to diagnosis of Morvan syndrome relies on the recognition of simultaneous PNS and CNS involvement (nearly all have neuromyotonia and neuropsychiatric disturbances), supported heavily by EDX findings of PNH and supplemented by neural antibody testing. VGKC-complex antibodies are present in most (70%–90%), usually against Caspr2 but also LGI1, either alone or in combination.[39,42] Magnetic resonance imaging of the brain typically is normal, which can help discriminate Morvan from limbic encephalitis.[19,39,44] Spinal fluid abnormalities (unmatched oligoclonal bands or elevated protein levels) are present in fewer than half.[2] Autonomic testing (sweating and cardiovascular abnormalities) and polysomnography (lack of sleep architecture and loss of REM atonia) can be useful adjunctive tests. Tumors (41%), especially thymoma, and myasthenia gravis (31%) are common associations.[37,42] Up to a third of patients eventually may succumb to Morvan syndrome, much more commonly when in association with cancer.[37,42]

TREATMENT CONSIDERATIONS

Management of PMH largely has been informed by the experience of case reports and various case series. In general, those with minor symptoms limited to the PNS can be managed symptomatically whereas those with more severe peripheral disease or involvement of the CNS or ANS should be considered for immunotherapy.

Symptomatic treatment is helpful for the manifestations of PNH in most patients, regardless of underlying etiology. Drugs that stabilize neuronal membranes (antiepileptic drugs primarily) have been reported as most useful, including carbamazepine, phenytoin, and gabapentin, which have been reported to improve symptoms in a majority of patients.[1,45] Various case reports note the possible utility of oxcarbazepine, pregabalin, lamotrigine, mexiletine, acetazolamide, topiramate, and valproate (reviewed by Elangovan and colleagues[32]).

In those cases of a suspected autoimmune basis, immunotherapy often is necessary, and regimens are similar to those used for the autoimmune encephalitides (for a detailed review of treatment strategies for autoimmune neurologic conditions, see Linnoila and Pittock[46]). Steroids, intravenous immunoglobulins, and plasmapheresis commonly are employed to induce remission, either as monotherapies or in combination.[42,47,48] Although clinical presentation classically is subacute with clinical nadir by 4 months, patients still may respond to treatment despite prolonged symptom duration of months to years.[49] In refractory cases, escalation to second-line treatments (rituximab and cyclophosphamide) may be necessary.[47] Maintenance therapies have included mycophenolate mofetil and azathioprine.[42,47]

In the setting of Caspr2 antibodies, a good or full response to immunotherapy (with tumor treatment if necessary) can be expected in approximately half of patients, with the remainder experiencing either a partial (44%) or no response (7%).[47] In patients with LGI1 antibodies, first-line immunotherapies initially are effective in 80%, with up to 67% experiencing a favorable outcome.

DISCLOSURE

Drs S. Hutto and T.B. Harrison report no disclosures.

REFERENCES

1. Jamieson PW, Katirji MB. Idiopathic generalized myokymia. Muscle Nerve 1994; 17(1):42–51.
2. Hart IK, Maddison P, Newsom-Davis J, et al. Phenotypic variants of autoimmune peripheral nerve hyperexcitability. Brain 2002;125(Pt 8):1887–95.
3. Morvan AM. De la choree bibrillaire per de Dr Morvan de Lannills. Gaz Hebdomadaire de Med de Chirurgie 1890;27:173.
4. Serratrice G, Azulay JP. [What is left of Morvan's fibrillary chorea?]. Rev Neurol (Paris) 1994;150(4):257–65.
5. Isaacs H. A syndrome of continuous muscle-fibre activity. J Neurol Neurosurg Psychiatry 1961;24(4):319–25.
6. Tahmoush AJ, Alonso RJ, Tahmoush GP, et al. Cramp-fasciculation syndrome: a treatable hyperexcitable peripheral nerve disorder. Neurology 1991;41(7): 1021–4.
7. Ahmed A, Simmons Z. Isaacs syndrome: a review. Muscle Nerve 2015; 52(1):5–12.
8. Denny-Brown D, Pennybacker J. Fibrillation and fasciculations in voluntary muscle. Brain 1938;61:311–34.
9. Gutmann L, Gutmann L. Myokymia and neuromyotonia 2004. J Neurol 2004; 251(2):138–42.
10. Layzer RB. The origin of muscle fasciculations and cramps. Muscle Nerve 1994; 17(11):1243–9.
11. Miller TM, Layzer RB. Muscle cramps. Muscle Nerve 2005;32(4):431–42.
12. Dengler R, de Carvalho M, Shahrizaila N, et al. AANEM - IFCN glossary of terms in neuromuscular electrodiagnostic medicine and ultrasound. Clin Neurophysiol 2020;131(7):1662–3.
13. Denny-Brown D, Foley J. Myokymia and the benighn fasciculation of muscular cramps. Trans Assoc Am Physic 1948;61:88–96.
14. Auger RG. AAEM minimonograph #44: diseases associated with excess motor unit activity. Muscle Nerve 1994;17(11):1250–63.

15. Gutmann L. AAEM minimonograph #37: facial and limb myokymia. Muscle Nerve 1991;14(11):1043–9.
16. Sawlani K, Katirji B. Peripheral Nerve Hyperexcitability Syndromes. Continuum (Minneap Minn) 2017;23(5):1437–50.
17. Mertens HG, Zschocke S. [Neuromyotonia]. Klin Wochenschr 1965;43(17): 917–25.
18. Gutmann L, Libell D, Gutmann L. When is myokymia neuromyotonia? Muscle Nerve 2001;24(2):151–3.
19. Josephs KA, Silber MH, Fealey RD, et al. Neurophysiologic studies in Morvan syndrome. J Clin Neurophysiol 2004;21(6):440–5.
20. Niu J, Guan H, Cui L, et al. Afterdischarges following M waves in patients with voltage-gated potassium channels antibodies. Clin Neurophysiol Pract 2017; 2:72–5.
21. Rubio-Agusti I, Perez-Miralles F, Sevilla T, et al. Peripheral nerve hyperexcitability: a clinical and immunologic study of 38 patients. Neurology 2011;76(2):172–8.
22. Maddison P, Mills KR, Newsom-Davis J. Clinical electrophysiological characterization of the acquired neuromyotonia phenotype of autoimmune peripheral nerve hyperexcitability. Muscle Nerve 2006;33(6):801–8.
23. Auger RG, Daube JR, Gomez MR, et al. Hereditary form of sustained muscle activity of peripheral nerve origin causing generalized myokymia and muscle stiffness. Ann Neurol 1984;15(1):13–21.
24. Nair AV, Mani A, Vijayaraghavan A, et al. Utility of stimulus induced after discharges in the evaluation of peripheral nerve hyperexcitability: old wine in a new bottle? J Peripher Nerv Syst 2021;26:90–8.
25. Harrison TB, Benatar M. Accuracy of repetitive nerve stimulation for diagnosis of the cramp-fasciculation syndrome. Muscle Nerve 2007;35(6):776–80.
26. Benatar M, Chapman KM, Rutkove SB. Repetitive nerve stimulation for the evaluation of peripheral nerve hyperexcitability. J Neurol Sci 2004;221(1–2):47–52.
27. Bodkin CL, Kennelly KD, Boylan KB, et al. Defining normal duration for afterdischarges with repetitive nerve stimulation: a pilot study. J Clin Neurophysiol 2009;26(1):45–9.
28. Liewluck T, Klein CJ, Jones LK Jr. Cramp-fasciculation syndrome in patients with and without neural autoantibodies. Muscle Nerve 2014;49(3):351–6.
29. Verdru P, Leenders J, Van Hees J. Cramp-fasciculation syndrome. Neurology 1992;42(9):1846–7.
30. Vernino S, Lennon VA. Ion channel and striational antibodies define a continuum of autoimmune neuromuscular hyperexcitability. Muscle Nerve 2002;26(5):702–7.
31. Vernino S, Auger RG, Emslie-Smith AM, et al. Myasthenia, thymoma, presynaptic antibodies, and a continuum of neuromuscular hyperexcitability. Neurology 1999; 53(6):1233–9.
32. Elangovan C, Morawo A, Ahmed A. Current treatment options for peripheral nerve hyperexcitability syndromes. Curr Treat Options Neurol 2018;20(7):23.
33. D'Adamo MC, Hasan S, Guglielmi L, et al. New insights into the pathogenesis and therapeutics of episodic ataxia type 1. Front Cell Neurosci 2015;9:317.
34. Peeters K, Chamova T, Tournev I, et al. Axonal neuropathy with neuromyotonia: there is a HINT. Brain 2017;140(4):868–77.
35. Kucukali CI, Kurtuncu M, Akcay HI, et al. Peripheral nerve hyperexcitability syndromes. Rev Neurosci 2015;26(2):239–51.
36. Newsom-Davis J, Mills KR. Immunological associations of acquired neuromyotonia (Isaacs' syndrome). Report of five cases and literature review. Brain 1993; 116(Pt 2):453–69.

37. Irani SR, Alexander S, Waters P, et al. Antibodies to Kv1 potassium channel-complex proteins leucine-rich, glioma inactivated 1 protein and contactin-associated protein-2 in limbic encephalitis, Morvan's syndrome and acquired neuromyotonia. Brain 2010;133(9):2734–48.

38. Montojo MT, Petit-Pedrol M, Graus F, et al. Clinical spectrum and diagnostic value of antibodies against the potassium channel related protein complex. Neurologia 2015;30(5):295–301.

39. Irani SR, Vincent A. Voltage-gated potassium channel-complex autoimmunity and associated clinical syndromes. Handb Clin Neurol 2016;133:185–97.

40. Bien CG, Vincent A, Barnett MH, et al. Immunopathology of autoantibody-associated encephalitides: clues for pathogenesis. Brain 2012;135(Pt 5): 1622–38.

41. Tomimitsu H, Arimura K, Nagado T, et al. Mechanism of action of voltage-gated K+ channel antibodies in acquired neuromyotonia. Ann Neurol 2004;56(3): 440–4.

42. Irani SR, Pettingill P, Kleopa KA, et al. Morvan syndrome: clinical and serological observations in 29 cases. Ann Neurol 2012;72(2):241–55.

43. Vincent A, Pettingill P, Pettingill R, et al. Association of leucine-rich glioma inactivated Protein 1, contactin-associated Protein 2, and Contactin 2 antibodies with clinical features and patient-reported pain in acquired neuromyotonia. JAMA Neurol 2018;75(12):1519–27.

44. Cortelli P, Perani D, Montagna P, et al. Pre-symptomatic diagnosis in fatal familial insomnia: serial neurophysiological and 18FDG-PET studies. Brain 2006;129(Pt 3):668–75.

45. Hurst RL, Hobson-Webb LD. Therapeutic implications of peripheral nerve hyperexcitability in muscle cramping: a retrospective review. J Clin Neurophysiol 2016; 33(6):560–3.

46. Linnoila J, Pittock SJ. Autoantibody-associated central nervous system neurologic disorders. Semin Neurol 2016;36(4):382–96.

47. van Sonderen A, Arino H, Petit-Pedrol M, et al. The clinical spectrum of Caspr2 antibody-associated disease. Neurology 2016;87(5):521–8.

48. van Sonderen A, Thijs RD, Coenders EC, et al. Anti-LGI1 encephalitis: clinical syndrome and long-term follow-up. Neurology 2016;87(14):1449–56.

49. Merchut MP. Management of voltage-gated potassium channel antibody disorders. Neurol Clin 2010;28(4):941–59.

Electromyography Case Examples

Practical Approaches to Neuromuscular Symptoms

Christopher J. Lamb, MD*, Devon I. Rubin, MD

KEYWORDS

- Electromyography • Nerve conduction studies • Decision-making • Diagnosis
- Neuromuscular disorders

KEY POINTS

- The choice of nerve conduction studies and muscles examined with electromyography should be individualized to each patient based on the history and examination.
- Examiners should prepare by considering all of the possible localizations of the patient's complaint before beginning to help decide each test, and the interpretation of the findings.
- Each nerve conduction performed or muscle chosen for electromyography should have a specific goal and rationale, providing useful information even if the result is normal.

INTRODUCTION

Many neuromuscular complaints are evaluated with electrodiagnostic (EDX) testing. In practice, physicians must plan the EDX study to provide the most useful information addressing patients' symptoms. The approach to each study must be individualized based on the symptoms and findings of each previous result. This article reviews EDX approaches, rationale, and findings for five actual patients. The goal is to provide rationale for why specific studies were selected and how each was helpful in deriving the final diagnosis.

CASE 1: A GARDENER WITH BACK AND LEG PAIN

A 68-year-old man described burning pain and paresthesia from his feet to his hips slowly intensifying over 6 months while he worked in his garden. The pain was worst at night. He also had worsening chronic low back pain beginning 15 years prior. His legs fatigued after standing or walking for 5 to 10 minutes. Examination revealed

Department of Neurology, Mayo Clinic, 4500 San Pablo Road South, Jacksonville, FL 32224, USA
* Corresponding author.
E-mail address: lamb.christopher@mayo.edu

Neurol Clin 39 (2021) 1097–1111
https://doi.org/10.1016/j.ncl.2021.06.010   **neurologic.theclinics.com**
0733-8619/21/© 2021 Elsevier Inc. All rights reserved.

preserved strength, hyporeflexia at the knees and ankles, and reduced pinprick sensation in both feet to the midcalves. He had difficulty walking on his heels and toes.

Differential Diagnosis

Slowly progressive "burning" feet are often the initial presentation of polyneuropathy. Low back pain is common in the general population and may be not be neurologic; however, the patient's leg symptoms in the context of back pain could be caused by multiple lumbosacral radiculopathies (especially L5/S1). Because radiculopathies and polyneuropathies are common, both conditions could be present. A diffuse poly-radiculoneuropathy or bilateral lumbosacral plexopathies were less likely.

Electrodiagnostic Findings and Interpretation

Nerve conduction studies (NCS) and needle electromyography (EMG) findings are shown in **Tables 1** and **2**. These findings were consistent with a chronic, length-dependent, axonal, sensorimotor peripheral neuropathy. There was no electrophysiologic evidence of a right lumbosacral radiculopathy.

Electrodiagnostic Approach and Case Discussion

"Burning feet" has several potential neurologic causes, the most likely being a length-dependent polyneuropathy. The goal of the EDX study in this case was to evaluate for polyneuropathy, lumbosacral radiculopathies, or a polyradiculopathy. The patient's clinical features suggested sensory more than motor fiber involvement; however, the fibular and tibial motor NCS were performed to assess for subclinical axonal loss or demyelination of the distal motor fibers. Although low fibular and tibial compound muscle action potential (CMAP) and slowed conduction velocity (CV) could be consistent with a distal polyneuropathy, similar changes may occur from long-standing L5/S1 radiculopathies or polyradiculopathy. Fibular and tibial F waves assessed the proximal nerve segment. Disproportionate slowing of F waves compared with the distal segment would have supported polyradiculopathy. Although prolonged F wave latencies may sometimes occur with single root lesions, F waves have low sensitivity in lumbosacral radiculopathies.[1] In this case, F wave latencies fell within estimates, which argues against a polyradiculopathy.

Sural sensory nerve action potential (SNAP) may be absent in older patients without disease, limiting the interpretation of this finding. They are performed to assess the distal, postganglionic sensory axons, especially because the primary complaint is sensory. Normal lower limb SNAPs support sparing of large sensory fibers distal to

Table 1
Case 1 nerve conduction study findings

Stimulate (Record)	Amplitude (mV or μV)			Conduction Velocity (m/s)			Distal Latency (ms)			F Wave Latency (ms)		
	R	L	NL	R	L	NL	R	L	NL	R	L	EST
Fibular, m (ext. dig. brevis)	**2.0**		>2	**39**		>41	3.1		<4.5	61.7		66.7
Tibial, m (abd. Hal.)	**2.1**		>4	**38**		>40	3.7		<6.1	62.1		67.3
Sural, s (malleolus)	**NR**		NR			>40	**NR**		<4.5			
Ulnar, m (hypothenar)	10.7		>6	**49**		>51	2.9		<3.6			
Median, s anti (index)	11		>15	**54**		>56	3.3		<3.6			

Bolded values are abnormal.
Abbreviations: EST, F wave latency estimate; NL, normal values; NR, No response.

Table 2
Case 1 needle electromyography findings

Muscle	Insertional Activity	Fibrillation Potentials	MUP	Recruitment	Duration	Amplitude	% Polyphasic
Gluteus maximus	NL	0	NL				
Tensor fasciae latae	NL	0	NL				
Vastus medialis	NL	0	NL				
GastrocnemiMUP, motor unit potential; us (medial head)	Increased	1+		NL	1+ long	1+ high	
Tibialis anterior	NL	0	Unstable	NL	1+ long		25

Bolded values are abnormal.
Abbreviation: MUP, motor unit potential; NL, normal.

the dorsal root ganglion. Despite this, values falling within "normal" reference range (eg, 9 μV amplitude) may be reduced for any individual patient, because any individual's own "normal" value is often unknown.

Because all lower limb NCS responses were abnormal in this patient, NCS were extended to the clinically unaffected upper limb. The low median SNAP and slowed upper limb conduction velocities supported a more diffuse polyneuropathy, although similar findings could also be seen in polyradiculoneuropathy. Furthermore, a concomitant lumbosacral radiculopathy with a superimposed distal polyneuropathy cannot be excluded based on NCS alone, making needle EMG necessary.

Needle EMG demonstrated chronic neurogenic findings in distal leg muscles, which could be seen in length-dependent polyneuropathy, L5/S1 radiculopathies, or both, necessitating EMG of proximal L5- and S1-innervated muscles. Normal needle EMG findings in proximal muscles with the same root innervations argued against multiple radiculopathies or a polyradiculopathy, and further supported length-dependent polyneuropathy.

The EDX findings in this case supported the diagnosis of a length-dependent, axonal polyneuropathy involving large motor and sensory fibers. The distinction between a primarily axonal or demyelinating neuropathy has important implications for management. EDX criteria for demyelination should be used in the interpretation of the study.[2] In this case, normal distal latencies, minimal CV slowing in the context of reduced CMAP amplitudes, normal F waves, and lack of abnormal temporal dispersion confirmed a predominantly axonal neuropathy.

Clinics Care Points

- "Burning feet" are frequently caused by polyneuropathy, but could occur in L5/S1 radiculopathies, polyradiculoneuropathy, or myelopathy.
- Needle examination of proximal L5 and S1 muscles is important to help distinguish a length-dependent polyneuropathy from lumbosacral radiculopathies or a polyradiculopathy.
- Axonal neuropathies are characterized by predominantly decreased CMAP and SNAP amplitudes, although mild slowing of CV often occurs because of loss of some of the fastest conducting axons.

CASE 2: A HAIRDRESSER WITH PAINLESS LEFT ARM WEAKNESS

A 48-year-old hairdresser developed painless left-hand weakness over 1 year. She wore a wrist brace for several months for presumed carpal tunnel syndrome. Left carpal and cubital tunnel release, followed by C5-C7 anterior cervical discectomy and fusion, provided no benefit, and weakness of her proximal left arm and distal right arm progressed.

Examination demonstrated left hand and forearm atrophy; severe weakness of left shoulder abduction; elbow flexion and extension; digit abduction, extension, and flexion; and complete left wrist drop. There was mild weakness of neck flexion, right elbow and wrist extension, and right digit abduction. Reflexes were asymmetrically brisk in upper more than lower limbs. Tone was increased in her left more than right upper limbs. Fasciculations were visible in the left deltoid and quadriceps muscles.

Differential Diagnosis

Painless, progressive, asymmetric weakness with upper (UMN) and lower motor neuron (LMN) signs is most concerning for motor neuron disease (MND), such as amyotrophic lateral sclerosis (ALS). Cervical myelopathy may account for some UMN findings. Painless wrist drop, along with weakness in multiple nerve distributions raises the possibility of multifocal motor neuropathy with conduction block (MMN-CB), although hyperreflexia is not typical. A patchy polyradiculoneuropathy, multiple mono-neuropathies, or asymmetric myopathy superimposed on cervical myelopathy could also be considered.

Electrodiagnostic Summary and Interpretation

NCS are shown in **Table 3**. There was no evidence of conduction block (CB), abnormal temporal dispersion, or focal slowing between distal and proximal sites in any motor nerve. EMG is summarized in **Table 4**. The findings were interpreted as showing evidence consistent with a diffuse, progressive MND, such as could be seen with ALS.

Electrodiagnostic Approach and Discussion

The goals of NCS in patients with possible MND are to (1) establish evidence of motor axonal loss; (2) confirm sparing of sensory axons; and (3) evaluate for the presence of mimickers, such as motor-predominant polyradiculopathy or MMN-CB. NCS selection depends on the distribution of clinical involvement; at least one motor and sensory NCS should be performed in each affected limb. In some cases, more NCS are necessary to thoroughly assess for patchy or asymmetric temporal dispersion or CB. The radial motor NCS was performed to assess for focal CB because radial muscles were clinically severely weak. Radial CMAP amplitudes were low at both stimulation sites without CB. Radial muscle weakness with normal elbow (distal) and spiral groove amplitudes would have prompted more proximal stimulation at the axilla and/or supra-clavicular fossa to evaluate for CB. Several motor and sensory NCS were performed in the lower limbs to assess for subtle involvement of lower limbs, which may also be useful as baseline values for future comparison.

The approach to needle EMG in suspected MND involves the examination of multiple muscles with different innervations in lumbosacral, thoracic, cervical, and/or bulbar segments. The diagnosis of MND is supported by abnormalities in two to three muscles in three contiguous segments and exclusion of alternative diagnoses.[3,4] Fibrillations, reduced recruitment, and long duration, high amplitude motor unit potential (MUP) may be obvious in atrophied or weak muscles, but attention should be paid to muscles that are not clinically affected for early signs of axonal involvement, such as fasciculations or MUP instability.[3] Although there were no clinically evident LMN signs or

Table 3
Case 2 nerve conduction studies

Stimulate (Record)	Amplitude (mV or μV)			Conduction Velocity (m/s)			Distal Latency (ms)		
	R	L	NL	R	L	NL	R	L	NL
Ulnar, m (hypothenar)		1.2	>6		53	>51		2.3	<3.6
Ulnar, s anti (fifth)		34	>10		57	>54		2.4	<3.1
Median, m (thenar)		0.5	>4		46	>48		2.8	<4.5
Median, s anti (index)		38	>15		61	>56		2.8	<3.6
Radial, m (EDC)		0.2			63	>67		2.9	<3.1
Fibular, m (ext. dig. brevis)		4.3	>2		53	>41		3.6	<4.5
Tibial, m (abd. hal.)		13.4	>4		52	>40		3.8	<6.1
Sural, s (ankle)		10	>6		49	>40		3.5	<4.5

Bolded values are abnormal.
Abbreviation: EDC, extensor digitorum communis; NL, normal values.

Table 4
Case 2 electromyography findings

Muscle	Side	Insertional Activity	Fibrillations	Fasciculations	MUP	Recruitment	Duration	Amplitude	% Polyphasic
First dorsal interosseous	L	Increased	3+	0	None				
Extensor indicis proprius	L	Increased	3+	0	None				
Pronator teres	L	Increased	3+	0	Unstable	Reduced 1+	3+ long	2+ high	100
Biceps brachii	L	Increased	2+	0	Unstable		1+ long	1+ high	50
Triceps brachii	L	Increased	2+	0	Unstable				50
C8 paraspinal	L	Increased	1+	1+	NL				
T4 paraspinal	L	NL	0	2+					
T10 paraspinal	L	Increased	2+	0			1+ long	1+ high	25
Tensor fasciae lata	L	Increased	1+	0	Unstable		1+ long	1+ high	25
Vastus medialis	L	Increased	1+	0	NL				
Gastrocnemius (medial)	L	Increased	0	1+	NL				
Tibialis anterior	L	NL	0	0	NL				

Bolded values are abnormal.
Abbreviation: NL, normal.

symptoms in the lower limbs, fibrillation potentials and unstable MUPs were present, providing evidence of early, widespread motor neuron involvement.

Other considerations, such as polyradiculoneuropathy, multiple mononeuropathies, MMN-CB, and myopathy, were excluded with normal SNAPs and absence of CBs and myopathic MUP changes. Although similar EDX findings are seen in motor-predominant axonal polyradiculopathies, these are typically associated with sensory symptoms and reduced deep tendon reflexes. In cases where polyneuropathy is superimposed on MND, SNAP responses may be abnormal, posing a challenge in the interpretation of the EDX data. Exclusion of demyelination and confirmation of motor neurogenic findings outside the distribution of sensory loss (eg, proximal and paraspinal muscles) increases confidence in MND diagnosis. If sensory loss is severe and unusual for polyneuropathy, the possibility of polyradiculoneuropathy may remain.

Long-standing myopathies, such as inclusion body myositis, may mimic MND because of the presence of widespread clinical weakness and atrophy coupled with the presence of myopathic and neurogenic EMG findings.[5] Disease duration, distribution, progression, and presence or absence of UMN signs are helpful clinical distinctions. Examiners should pay attention to myopathic MUPs, which may be overlooked among larger neurogenic MUPs.

Clinics Care Points

- Electrodiagnosis of ALS is supported by ongoing motor axonal loss in two muscles with differing innervation in $\geq$3 contiguous segments of the neuroaxis.
- The presence of CB on NCS, or the presence of abnormal sensory NCS responses is atypical for MND, and raises the possibility of MMN-CB or a polyradiculoneuropathy.
- Early signs of axonal loss (eg, motor unit instability) may be present on needle EMG in muscles that are not clinically affected.

CASE 3: A 24-YEAR-OLD MOTHER WITH PROGRESSIVE PROXIMAL MUSCLE WEAKNESS

A 24-year-old mother was referred for 3 years of slowly progressive proximal muscle weakness. She gradually lost the ability to climb stairs or reach above her head and, transitioned to a power chair because of exertional dyspnea and heart failure. Creatine kinase (CK) was 954 U/L, and troponin T was mildly elevated. Examination revealed large calf muscles and weakness of proximal more than distal, lower more than upper limb muscles, including shoulder abduction, elbow extension, hip flexion, knee extension and flexion, ankle dorsiflexion and plantarflexion. Reflexes were reduced in the upper limbs and absent in the lower limbs. There was no clinical myotonia.

Differential Diagnosis

Painless, progressive, symmetric, and proximal muscle weakness with hyporeflexia suggests several possibilities including myopathy, LMN-predominant MND, motor-predominant polyradiculoneuropathy, or neuromuscular junction (NMJ) disorder. Elevated CK increases likelihood of myopathy; however, CK may also be elevated in MND or axonal neuropathies.

Electrodiagnostic Summary and Interpretation

Right arm and leg NCS were normal (**Table 5**). EMG findings are shown in **Table 6**. These findings were consistent with a chronic, proximal myopathy characterized by fibrillations and myotonic discharges.

Table 5 Case 3 nerve conduction studies									
	Amplitude (mV or μV)			Conduction Velocity (m/s)			Distal Latency (ms)		
Stimulate (Record)	R	L	NL	R	L	NL	R	L	NL
Ulnar, m (hypothenar)	9.9		>6	73		>51	2.3		<3.6
Median, s anti (index)	58		>15	73		>56	2.5		<3.6
Fibular, m (ext. dig. brevis)	3.0		>2	57		>41	2.6		<4.5
Medial plantar, s (malleolus)	21		>7				2.4		<4.0

Abbreviation: NL, normal values.

Electrodiagnostic Approach and Discussion

The EDX approach to patients who present with symmetric, proximal weakness includes a combination of NCS, EMG, and often repetitive nerve stimulation (RNS). Although most EDX studies begin with NCS, performing needle EMG first occasionally helps to decrease the number of necessary NCS. If prominent neurogenic or myopathic changes are found on EMG, RNS may be unnecessary.

Routine motor NCS (distal legs and arms) may be normal when weakness is predominantly proximal. However, CMAP amplitudes may be low in patients with distal or severe, generalized myopathies. Low amplitudes and/or slowed CVs are seen in overlapping myopathy and neuropathy, or in other diagnoses, such as a polyradiculoneuropathy. When weakness is symmetric and proximal, at least one motor and sensory NCS is performed in the most affected limbs. Additional NCS are performed when suspicion for nonmyopathic conditions is higher. If the suspicion for NMJ disorder is high, RNS should be performed on a distal and proximal muscle.

The primary goals of needle EMG in the evaluation of a suspected myopathy are to (1) confirm its presence by demonstrating myopathic findings; (2) identify pattern of involvement (proximal and/or distal); (3) characterize the myopathy (eg, fibrillations, myotonic discharges); and (4) identify a muscle suitable for biopsy, if indicated. If biopsy is considered, EMG should be performed unilaterally to spare the contralateral muscle from needle insertion artifact on biopsy. EMG should focus on clinically affected muscles including proximal and distal muscles in leg, arm, and paraspinals. The paraspinal muscles may be the earliest or only muscles involved in mild inflammatory myopathies, adult-onset acid-maltase deficiency,[6] or systemic amyloidosis.[7]

Although EMG often does not provide a specific cause, it may narrow the differential diagnoses of genetic, inflammatory, and infectious myopathies. Fibrillations indicate the presence of pathologic changes, such as muscle fiber splitting, necrosis, or vacuolar damage.[8] Myotonic discharges may be seen in various myopathies but, when diffuse, they suggest a myotonic disorder, some dystrophies, or acid-maltase deficiency. Diffuse myotonic discharges without weakness or abnormal MUPs may suggest myotonia congenita, in which there is usually prominent percussion myotonia. Myopathic MUPs have short duration, low amplitude, polyphasia, and early/rapid recruitment. Confidence in myopathy diagnosis is greatly increased by the presence of greater than one myopathic finding (eg, fibrillations + short-duration MUPs + rapid recruitment).

This patient demonstrated EDX findings consistent with a proximal myopathy. The fibrillation potentials and myotonic discharges raised the possibility of an inherited or inflammatory myopathy. Genetic testing later revealed a pathogenic autosomal-dominant Lamin A/C gene mutation consistent with Emery-Dreifuss muscular dystrophy type 2.

Table 6
Case 3 electromyography findings

Muscle	Side	Insertional Activity	Fibrillation Potentials	MUP	Recruitment	Duration	Amplitude	% Polyphasic
Deltoid	R	Increased	3+		2+ rapid	2+ short	2+ low	75
Biceps	R	Increased	2+		2+ rapid	2+ short	2+ low	50
First dorsal interosseous	R	Increased	1+	NL				
Ext digitorum communis	R	Increased	2+		2+ rapid	1+ short	1+ low	25
Triceps	R	Increased	3+		1+ rapid			50
Vastus medialis	R	Increased	2+		1+ rapid	2+ short	2+ low	25
Iliopsoas	R	Increased	3+		2+ rapid	2+ short	2+ low	100
Tibialis anterior	R	Increased	3+		2+ rapid	2+ short	1+ low	75
Medial gastrocnemius	R	Increased	2+			1+ short		
T10 paraspinal	R	Increased	2+	0	3+ rapid			75
Myotonic discharges were present in all muscles examined								

Abbreviation: NL, normal.

Clinics Care Points

- Painless, symmetric, proximal weakness should raise suspicion of myopathy, although NMJ disorders, polyradiculopathies, or motor neuron disorders can present similarly.
- Needle EMG is the most sensitive EDX test for myopathy and can help (1) to confirm the presence; (2) characterize the nature, chronicity, distribution; and (3) identify the appropriate muscle for biopsy.
- Examining clinically weak and proximal muscles, including thoracic paraspinal muscles, cautiously listening for slow fibrillation potentials, and carefully assessing MUP recruitment and morphology are necessary to confirm mild myopathies.

CASE 4: A NAVAL VETERAN WITH HAND NUMBNESS

An 89-year-old retired naval veteran developed paresthesia of his left fourth and fifth digits over 5 years. With elbow flexion, the paresthesia of his left fourth and fifth digits became more intense and occasionally awoke him from sleep. He had mild hand pain while sleeping. His neurologic examination revealed normal objective sensory testing of the upper and lower limbs to pin and light touch, and normal strength and reflexes.

Differential Diagnosis

The patient's clinical history and distribution of symptoms suggests a left ulnar mononeuropathy, although a left lower trunk brachial plexopathy or C8/T1 radiculopathies could also cause similar symptoms.

Electrodiagnostic Summary and Interpretation

Left upper limb NCS are shown in **Table 7**. Short segmental stimulation study ("inching") of left ulnar sensory response revealed a focal latency shift of 1.2 milliseconds at a segment adjacent to the medial epicondyle, without CB. The left dorsal ulnar cutaneous (DUC) response was absent and the right DUC response was elicited with radial stimulation only, a normal anatomic variant.[9] EMG findings are shown in **Table 8**. These findings were consistent with mild left ulnar mononeuropathy at the elbow involving predominantly sensory fibers.

Electrodiagnostic Approach and Discussion

The approach to a patient with focal sensory symptoms in an arm or hand includes a combination of motor and sensory NCS and needle EMG. NCS are necessary to

---

Table 7
Case 4 nerve conduction studies

Stimulate (Record)	Amplitude (mV or μV)			Conduction Velocity (m/s)			Distal Latency (ms)		
	R	L	NL	R	L	NL	R	L	NL
Ulnar, m (hypothenar)		10.0	>6		53	>51		2.6	<3.6
Ulnar, s anti (fifth)		16	>10			>54		1.8	<3.1
Median, m (thenar)		8.5	>4		52	>48		4.1	<4.5
Median, s anti (index)		80	>15		57	>56		2.0	<3.6
Ulnar, s dorsal hand anti	3 (radial stimulation)	NR					3.3	NR	

Abbreviations: NL, normal values.

Table 8						
Case 4 electromyography findings						
Muscle	**Side**	**Insertional Activity**	**Fibrillation Potentials**	**MUP**	**Recruitment**	**Duration**
Deltoid	L	NL	0	NL		
Triceps	L	NL	0	NL		
First dorsal interosseous	L	NL	0		NL	1+ long
Flexor digitorum profundus III/IV	L	NL	0	NL		
Pronator teres	L	NL	0	NL		

Abbreviation: NL, normal.

assess multiple different individual nerves, to determine the presence of focal demyelination or axonal loss within one or more nerve distributions, and to help localize the area of injury at a specific site along the nerve. This patient's symptoms were isolated to the fourth and fifth digits, so the focus was on the ulnar nerve. Median NCS were also performed to screen for a more diffuse process (eg, a brachial plexopathy or polyneuropathy). If the median NCS were abnormal or if there was a higher level of suspicion of a lower trunk or medial cord brachial plexopathy, the medial antebrachial cutaneous nerve and other NCS would also have been considered.

The sensory fibers are often first to be involved in compressive mononeuropathies, but motor fibers are also evaluated, especially when patients have weakness. Furthermore, motor NCS are often better at detecting focal slowing or CB at a precise site along the nerve (eg, retrocondylar groove) than sensory NCS. When segmental slowing or CB is identified between the below and above elbow sites, lesions are more precisely localized using short segmental stimulation studies ("inching"). A 10 m/s difference in CV between above and below elbow segments, or above elbow CV less than 50 m/s should prompt an "inching" study, although a high level of suspicion is also sufficient.[10] A CMAP amplitude decrease of 10% or latency shift of greater than 0.8 milliseconds over 2 cm is evidence of focal demyelination.[11] Although "inching" is most often performed with motor NCS, it can also be used with ulnar sensory NCS when motor NCS are normal.[12]

The DUC sensory NCS can sometimes assist with ulnar neuropathy localization. The DUC branches from the ulnar nerve before entering Guyon canal in the wrist and it is spared in ulnar mononeuropathies at the wrist. If the response is abnormal, the localization would be expected to be at the elbow. Because the dorsal ulnar area of the hand is innervated by the superficial radial nerve in 16% of patients, stimulation of the superficial radial nerve at the forearm should be performed when the DUC is absent or low.[9]

Needle examination focused primarily on C8-T1 and ulnar-innervated muscles. Mild EMG abnormalities may be detected even if motor NCS responses are normal in some chronic, indolent processes where the pace of reinnervation equals that of denervation. EMG abnormalities in ulnar-innervated forearm muscles (eg, flexor carpi ulnaris or flexor digitorum profundus) in the absence of abnormalities in other nonulnar, C8 innervated muscles supports localization proximal to the forearm. However, these muscles may be spared in ulnar neuropathies at the retrocondylar groove or cubital tunnel.[13]

Although not performed in this patient, ultrasound evaluation of ulnar mononeuropathy may be performed to identify areas of focal nerve enlargement around the epicondylar groove when there is nonfocal slowing on ulnar NCS.[14]

Clinics Care Points

- Motor NCS, sensory NCS, and needle EMG are required to localize and assess ulnar mononeuropathy.
- Mild ulnar mononeuropathies predominantly involving sensory fibers may be further characterized using short segmental stimulation ("inching") study of the ulnar antidromic sensory NCS to evaluate for a definite latency shift between sites of stimulation.
- The DUC sensory response is useful to localize ulnar mononeuropathy.

CASE 5: A LONGSHOREMAN WITH HAND AND ARM PAIN

A 64-year-old retired, longshoreman with diabetes developed numbness, tingling, and pain in his hands and arms 6 months after cervical fusion for chronic neck pain. Paresthesia of bilateral digits I-IV awoke him from sleep. Such tasks as turning the key in the ignition, buttoning his shirt, and opening jars became more difficult.

Examination revealed bilateral thenar atrophy and thumb abduction, opposition, and digit extension weakness. Pinprick sensation was decreased over digits I-IV with sparing of the thenar eminence. The right biceps reflex was mildly diminished and there was mild, symmetric lower limb hyperreflexia.

Differential Diagnosis

This patient's hand paresthesia and pain could be related to several localizations. Although history and examination suggest features of an old cervical myelopathy, thenar atrophy and weakness and the distribution of his abnormal sensory examination are compatible with bilateral median mononeuropathies, bilateral cervical radiculopathies (C6-T1), or middle and lower trunk brachial plexopathies.

Electrodiagnostic Summary and Interpretation

Tables 9 and **10** display the patient's NCS and EMG findings. These findings were consistent with moderately severe median neuropathies at both wrists, consistent with carpal tunnel syndrome.

Electrodiagnostic Approach and Discussion

The goals of EDX testing in this patient were to localize the process to the median nerve, cervical roots, or both, and assess for an "active" process (vs residua of an

Table 9									
Case 5 nerve conduction studies									
	Amplitude (mV or μV)			**Conduction Velocity (m/s)**			**Distal Latency (ms)**		
Stimulate (Record)	R	L	NL	R	L	NL	R	L	NL
Ulnar, m (hypothenar)		8.7	>6		52	>51		2.6	<3.6
Ulnar, s anti (fifth)		11	>10		58	>54		2.9	<3.1
Median, m (thenar)	**4.0**	5.1	>4	49	**47**	>48	**10.5**	11.6	<4.5
Median, s anti (index)	NR	NR	>15	NR	NR	>56	NR	NR	<3.6

Bolded values are abnormal.
Abbreviation: NL, normal values.

Table 10
Case 5 needle electromyography findings

Muscle	Side	Insertional Activity	Fibrillation Potentials	MUP	Duration	Amplitude	% Polyphasic
Abductor pollicis brevis	L	NL	0		1+ long	1+ high	25
Biceps	L	NL	0	NL			
First dorsal interosseous	L	NL	0	NL			
Deltoid	L	NL	0	NL			
Triceps	L	NL	0	NL			
Pronator teres	L	NL	0	NL			
Extensor indicis proprius	L	NL	0	NL			

Abbreviation: NL, normal.

old, remote process) involving the cervical roots. Multiple superimposed peripheral nervous system conditions are common in practice, making interpretation of EDX findings more challenging.

Because this patient's symptoms and signs were bilateral, the most symptomatic limb was initially selected for NCS. Both median and ulnar motor and sensory studies also assess C8-T1 root levels and the lower trunk, except for the median antidromic sensory NCS, which assesses the upper trunk in 30% or middle trunk in 70% of patients.[15] The median motor study demonstrated a markedly prolonged distal latency, indicating severe demyelination in the distal segment of the median nerve, consistent with carpal tunnel syndrome. The ulnar motor NCS was performed to assess for diffuse demyelinating neuropathy or multiple mononeuropathies and was normal.

Because the median motor NCS was markedly abnormal, antidromic sensory studies were performed. If symptoms were mild, intermittent, or the median motor responses were normal, orthodromic (palmar) sensory studies would have been selected to increase sensitivity.

Although NCS indicated a severe median neuropathy at the wrist, given the patient's history of cervical spine disease and the possibility of superimposed cervical radiculopathies, needle EMG screened muscles supplied by C5-T1 roots. These were all normal, except abductor pollicis brevis (APB), thereby excluding active cervical radiculopathies.

Electrophysiologic severity of median neuropathy at the wrist does not always correlate with clinical symptoms but is useful to determine extent of nerve injury. Electrophysiologic grading of median neuropathy at the wrist varies by laboratory. Levels of severity are often based on the degree of involvement of sensory and motor fibers, with an expected progression beginning with prolonged distal latency of median sensory responses, progressing to decreased or absent median sensory responses (mild), then prolonged motor distal latency (moderate), and finally decreased motor amplitude or abnormal median MUPs on needle examination (severe).[16] This progression of abnormalities in electrophysiologic responses is a reflection of the natural history of focal compression and nerve injury over time beginning with focal demyelination at the site of compression of the more superficial sensory fibers, and gradually including more sensory and then motor fibers, represented by loss of SNAP and CMAP amplitude and MUP abnormalities.

Clinics Care Points

- Median neuropathy at the wrist EDX relies on identifying prolonged median distal latencies, with or without slow CV or low amplitude across the wrist.
- Electrophysiologic severity of median neuropathy at the wrist is estimated based on the pattern of involvement of sensory and motor distal latencies and amplitudes, along with any EMG changes in median-innervated thenar muscles.

SUMMARY

These cases represent typical patients and challenges faced by EDX physicians and technologists. They help to demonstrate a logical rationale for each decision and strategy when selecting studies during the EDX examination. Although each patient's clinical features require individualized strategies to establish a diagnosis, these cases review some guiding principles that generally apply to all patients, including the rationale for selecting motor and sensory NCS and for muscle selection during routine EMG.

DISCLOSURE

The authors have nothing to disclose.

REFERENCES

1. Mauricio EA, Dimberg EL, Rubin DI. Utility of minimum F-wave latencies compared with F-estimates and absolute reference values in S1 radiculopathies: are they still needed? Muscle Nerve 2014;49(6):809–13.
2. JTFot EFNS, PNS T. European Federation of Neurological Societies/Peripheral Nerve Society Guideline on management of chronic inflammatory demyelinating polyradiculoneuropathy: report of a joint task force of the European Federation of Neurological Societies and the Peripheral Nerve Society–First Revision. J Peripher Nervous Syst 2010;15(1):1–9.
3. de Carvalho M, Dengler R, Eisen A, et al. Electrodiagnostic criteria for diagnosis of ALS. Clin Neurophysiol 2008;119(3):497–503.
4. Brooks BR, Miller RG, Swash M, et al. El Escorial revisited: revised criteria for the diagnosis of amyotrophic lateral sclerosis. Amyotroph Lateral Scler other Mot Neuron Disord 2000;1(5):293–9.
5. Joy JL, Oh SJ, Baysal AI. Electrophysiological spectrum of inclusion body myositis. Muscle Nerve 1990;13(10):949–51.
6. Kassardjian CD, Engel AG, Sorenson EJ. Electromyographic findings in 37 patients with adult-onset acid maltase deficiency. Muscle Nerve 2015;51(5):759–61.
7. Rubin DI, Hermann RC. Electrophysiologic findings in amyloid myopathy. Muscle Nerve 1999;22(3):355–9.
8. Sener U, Martinez-Thompson J, Laughlin RS, et al. Needle electromyography and histopathologic correlation in myopathies. Muscle Nerve 2019;59(3):315–20.
9. Leis AA, Wells KJ. Radial nerve cutaneous innervation to the ulnar dorsum of the hand. Clin Neurophysiol 2008;119(3):662–6.
10. Kincaid JC, Phillips LH, Daube JR. The evaluation of suspected ulnar neuropathy at the elbow: normal conduction study values. Arch Neurol 1986;43(1):44–7.
11. Azrieli Y, Weimer L, Lovelace R, et al. The utility of segmental nerve conduction studies in ulnar mononeuropathy at the elbow. Muscle Nerve 2003;27(1):46–50.
12. Vazquez do Campo R, Dimberg E, Rubin D. Short segment sensory nerve stimulation in suspected ulnar neuropathy at the elbow: a pilot study. Muscle Nerve 2019;59(1):125–9.

13. Campbell WW, Pridgeon RM, Riaz G, et al. Sparing of the flexor carpi ulnaris in ulnar neuropathy at the elbow. Muscle Nerve 1989;12(12):965-7.
14. Preston DC, Shapiro BE. Electromyography and neuromuscular disorders: clinical-electrophysiologic-ultrasound correlations. 4th ed. Philadelphia: Elsevier, Inc.; 2020.
15. Ferrante MA, Wilbourn AJ. The utility of various sensory nerve conduction responses in assessing brachial plexopathies. Muscle Nerve 1995;18(8):879-89.
16. Medicine AAoE, Neurology AAo, Medicine AAoP, et al. Practice parameter for electrodiagnostic studies in carpal tunnel syndrome: summary statement. Muscle Nerve 2002;25(6):918-22.

UNITED STATES POSTAL SERVICE ®

Statement of Ownership, Management, and Circulation
(All Periodicals Publications Except Requester Publications)

1. Publication Title	2. Publication Number	3. Filing Date
NEUROLOGIC CLINICS	000 – 712	9/18/2021

4. Issue Frequency	5. Number of Issues Published Annually	6. Annual Subscription Price
FEB, MAY, AUG, NOV	4	$333.00

7. Complete Mailing Address of Known Office of Publication (Not printer) (Street, city, county, state, and ZIP+4®)

ELSEVIER INC.
230 Park Avenue, Suite 800
New York, NY 10169

Contact Person
Malathi Samayan

Telephone (Include area code)
91-44-4299-4507

8. Complete Mailing Address of Headquarters or General Business Office of Publisher (Not printer)

ELSEVIER INC.
230 Park Avenue, Suite 800
New York, NY 10169

9. Full Names and Complete Mailing Addresses of Publisher, Editor, and Managing Editor (Do not leave blank)

Publisher (Name and complete mailing address)

DOLORES MELONI, ELSEVIER INC.
1600 JOHN F KENNEDY BLVD. SUITE 1800
PHILADELPHIA, PA 19103-2899

Editor (Name and complete mailing address)

STACY EASTMAN, ELSEVIER INC.
1600 JOHN F KENNEDY BLVD. SUITE 1800
PHILADELPHIA, PA 19103-2899

Managing Editor (Name and complete mailing address)

PATRICK MANLEY, ELSEVIER INC.
1600 JOHN F KENNEDY BLVD. SUITE 1800
PHILADELPHIA, PA 19103-2899

10. Owner (Do not leave blank. If the publication is owned by a corporation, give the name and address of the corporation immediately followed by the names and addresses of all stockholders owning or holding 1 percent or more of the total amount of stock. If not owned by a corporation, give the names and addresses of the individual owners. If owned by a partnership or other unincorporated firm, give its name and address as well as those of each individual owner. If the publication is published by a nonprofit organization, give its name and address.)

Full Name	Complete Mailing Address
WHOLLY OWNED SUBSIDIARY OF REED/ELSEVIER, US HOLDINGS	1600 JOHN F KENNEDY BLVD. SUITE 1800 PHILADELPHIA, PA 19103-2899

11. Known Bondholders, Mortgagees, and Other Security Holders Owning or Holding 1 Percent or More of Total Amount of Bonds, Mortgages, or Other Securities. If none, check box ▶ ☐ None

Full Name	Complete Mailing Address
N/A	

12. Tax Status (For completion by nonprofit organizations authorized to mail at nonprofit rates) (Check one)
The purpose, function, and nonprofit status of this organization and the exempt status for federal income tax purposes:
☒ Has Not Changed During Preceding 12 Months
☐ Has Changed During Preceding 12 Months (Publisher must submit explanation of change with this statement)

PS Form 3526, July 2014 [Page 1 of 4 (see instructions page 4)] PSN: 7530-01-000-9931 PRIVACY NOTICE: See our privacy policy on www.usps.com.

---

13. Publication Title	14. Issue Date for Circulation Data Below
NEUROLOGIC CLINICS	MAY 2021

15. Extent and Nature of Circulation			Average No. Copies Each Issue During Preceding 12 Months	No. Copies of Single Issue Published Nearest to Filing Date
a. Total Number of Copies (Net press run)			237	218
b. Paid Circulation (By Mail and Outside the Mail)	(1)	Mailed Outside-County Paid Subscriptions Stated on PS Form 3541 (Include paid distribution above nominal rate, advertiser's proof copies, and exchange copies)	119	111
	(2)	Mailed In-County Paid Subscriptions Stated on PS Form 3541 (Include paid distribution above nominal rate, advertiser's proof copies, and exchange copies)	0	0
	(3)	Paid Distribution Outside the Mails Including Sales Through Dealers and Carriers, Street Vendors, Counter Sales, and Other Paid Distribution Outside USPS®	74	65
	(4)	Paid Distribution by Other Classes of Mail Through the USPS (e.g., First-Class Mail®)	0	0
c. Total Paid Distribution (Sum of 15b (1), (2), (3), and (4))			193	176
d. Free or Nominal Rate Distribution (By Mail and Outside the Mail)	(1)	Free or Nominal Rate Outside-County Copies included on PS Form 3541	26	24
	(2)	Free or Nominal Rate In-County Copies Included on PS Form 3541	0	0
	(3)	Free or Nominal Rate Copies Mailed at Other Classes Through the USPS (e.g., First-Class Mail)	0	0
	(4)	Free or Nominal Rate Distribution Outside the Mail (Carriers or other means)	0	0
e. Total Free or Nominal Rate Distribution (Sum of 15d (1), (2), (3) and (4))			26	24
f. Total Distribution (Sum of 15c and 15e)			219	200
g. Copies not Distributed (See Instructions to Publishers #4 (page #3))			18	18
h. Total (Sum of 15f and g)			237	218
i. Percent Paid (15c divided by 15f times 100)			88.12%	88%

* If you are claiming electronic copies, go to line 16 on page 3. If you are not claiming electronic copies, skip to line 17 on page 3.

16. Electronic Copy Circulation		Average No. Copies Each Issue During Preceding 12 Months	No. Copies of Single Issue Published Nearest to Filing Date
a. Paid Electronic Copies	▶		
b. Total Paid Print Copies (Line 15c) + Paid Electronic Copies (Line 16a)	▶		
c. Total Print Distribution (Line 15f) + Paid Electronic Copies (Line 16a)	▶		
d. Percent Paid (Both Print & Electronic Copies) (16b divided by 16c × 100)	▶		

☒ I certify that 50% of all my distributed copies (electronic and print) are paid above a nominal price.

17. Publication of Statement of Ownership

☒ If the publication is a general publication, publication of this statement is required. Will be printed in the **NOVEMBER 2021** issue of this publication. ☐ Publication not required.

18. Signature and Title of Editor, Publisher, Business Manager, or Owner

Malathi Samayan - Distribution Controller

Malathi Samayan

Date
9/18/2021

I certify that all information furnished on this form is true and complete. I understand that anyone who furnishes false or misleading information on this form or who omits material or information requested on the form may be subject to criminal sanctions (including fines and imprisonment) and/or civil sanctions (including civil penalties).

PS Form **3526**, July 2014 (Page 3 of 4)

PRIVACY NOTICE: See our privacy policy on www.usps.com

Moving?

Make sure your subscription moves with you!

To notify us of your new address, find your **Clinics Account Number** (located on your mailing label above your name), and contact customer service at:

Email: journalscustomerservice-usa@elsevier.com

800-654-2452 (subscribers in the U.S. & Canada)
314-447-8871 (subscribers outside of the U.S. & Canada)

Fax number: 314-447-8029

Elsevier Health Sciences Division
Subscription Customer Service
3251 Riverport Lane
Maryland Heights, MO 63043

*To ensure uninterrupted delivery of your subscription, please notify us at least 4 weeks in advance of move.

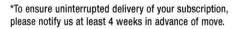

Printed and bound by CPI Group (UK) Ltd, Croydon, CR0 4YY

14/10/2024

01773715-0001